The Marfan Syndrome Patient's Sourcebook

Paul Kalman, MA

Johnson White, MD (Ed.)

© 2014 Paul Kalman, Johnson White

All Rights Reserved worldwide under the Berne Convention. May not be copied or distributed without prior written permission by the publisher.

ISBN 978-1499508802

Contents

INTRODUCTION 5

The Genetics of Marfan Syndrome 15

Signs and Symptoms 27

Diagnosis 55

Treatment 71

Pregnancy and MFS 123

Related disorders 127

Clinical Trials 137

Marfan Syndrome Related Organizations 139

GLOSSARY 143

REFERENCES 153

Index 161

INTRODUCTION

In 1896 Antoine Marfan, a French pediatrician, wrote about a five-year-old girl, named Gabrielle, who had abnormally slender fingers. He compared the girl's long fingers to spider legs (which is where the technical term for long fingers, "arachnodactyly" comes from). However, it wasn't until 1931 that another physician – Henricus Jacobus Marie Weve – coined the term "Marfan Syndrome" to describe a genetic disorder that affects the body's connective tissue. Marfan syndrome (MFS) can result in a myriad of signs and symptoms ranging from extremely long fingers to abnormalities with internal organs, including the heart.

"To some experts, Abraham Lincoln's long fingers and great height (he was 6'4") indicate that he may have suffered from [Marfan] syndrome. It has also been suggested that the long fingers that helped account for Niccolò Paganini's dexterity on the violin were the result of Marfan syndrome." (CNNSI)

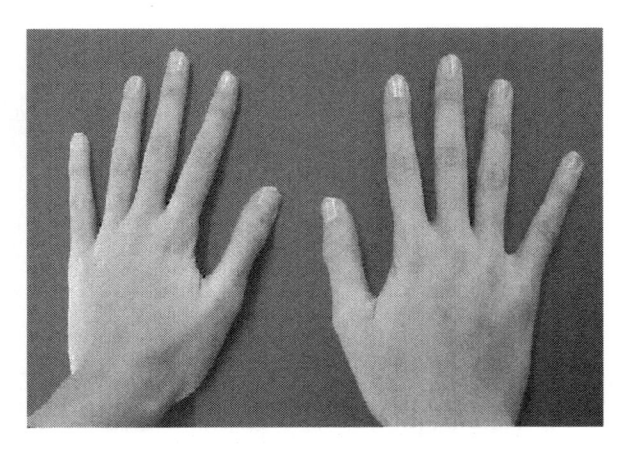

Arachnodactyly

Connective tissue holds all the organs, tissues and cells in your body together like glue. Because this tissue holds practically everything together, MFS can affect a nearly every system in your body. Although there are dozens of different ways MFS can affect you, the systems usually affected are the cardiovascular (heart and blood vessels) and ocular (eyes) along with the bones and joints.

Properly treated, and with careful monitoring, people with MFS can have a life-expectancy that's close to a person without MFS. However, it can be a life-threatening condition, even with treatment. For example, if the main blood vessel that carries blood away from the heart (the aorta) is dilated or if there is a bulge in the wall of the aorta (called a *thoracic aortic aneurysm*) this can result in early death.

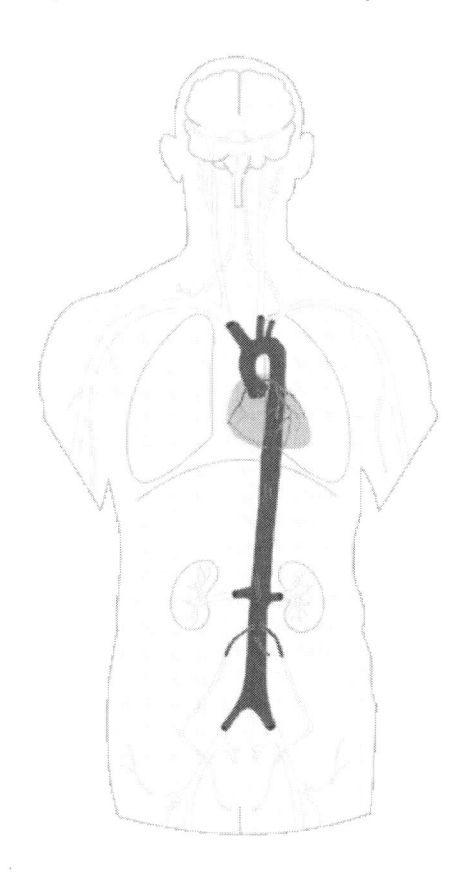

The Aorta

Improved detection and surgical techniques, and the use of beta-blockers to prevent heart complications all are helping to extend survival. The average lifespan for MFS patients is now about 70 years. If MFS is not treated, the average life expectancy is significantly reduced to 30-40 years (Chen).

In Marfan syndrome, there is usually a defect or mutation of the fibrillin-1 (FBN1) gene. The FBN1 gene tells the body how to make the fibrillin-1 protein. The fibrillin-1 protein is responsible for strengthening the body's connective tissue. This mutation causes the body to make too much of another protein called transforming growth factor beta (TGF-β), which results in problems with growth and development.

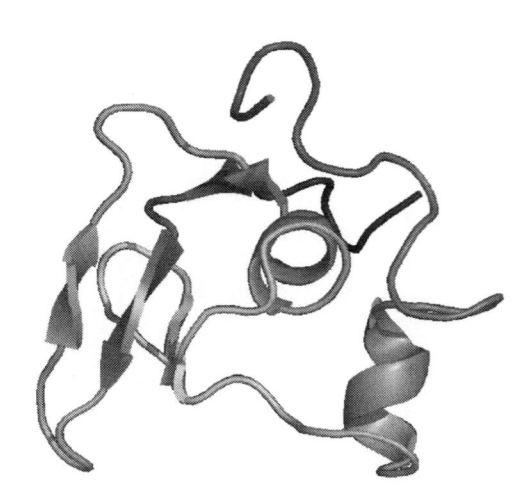

The FBN1 protein

Marfan syndrome is a genetic disease that runs in families. About 75% of people with Marfan syndrome inherit the disorder from their parents. The remaining 25% of patients are thought to have a spontaneous genetic mutation (Loeys et al. 2004, Liu et al. 2001, Turner et al. 2009).

Although FBN1 is the gene that most people think of being associated with MFS, not all MFS patients have a defect in FBN1. Misdiagnoses are not common, but they do happen. Some patients diagnosed with Marfan Syndrome may have mutations in another gene instead: either the TGFβR1 gene (Transforming Growth Factor-Beta Receptor, Type I) or the TGFβR2 gene (Transforming Growth Factor-Beta Receptor, Type II). If the TGFβR2 gene is affected, this used to be called Marfan syndrome Type II but (since 2006) is now called Loeys-Dietz syndrome. MFS and Loeys-Dietz are sometimes confused and misdiagnosed, especially if genetic testing is not carried out. Although the two syndromes manifest in very similar ways, dislocation of the lens of the eye and long fingers are not normally seen in Loeys-Dietz syndrome. However, Loeys-Dietz is a much more aggressive disorder that carries a very high risk of aortic aneurysms (bulges in the aorta) and premature death. It's therefore extremely important that you are diagnosed correctly. See the Related Disorders chapter for more information on Loeyz-Dietz.

"I was diagnosed with Marfan Syndrome in 2001. Ten years later, a doctor suspected I had a different connective tissue syndrome. A urine test was sent to the lab, and six weeks later I found out I didn't have MFS at all – it turns out I have a rare type of Ehler's Danlos. I'm still stunned that the correct diagnosis wasn't picked up all those years ago." Jill, Cheyenne Wyoming.

Abnormalities in either the *TGFβR2 or TGFβR1* genes are also associated with a Marfan-like syndrome that typically presents with aortic aneurysm and congenital abnormalities (Chen et. al). Which genes are affected can be identified with genetic testing, although testing is expensive and not 100% accurate.

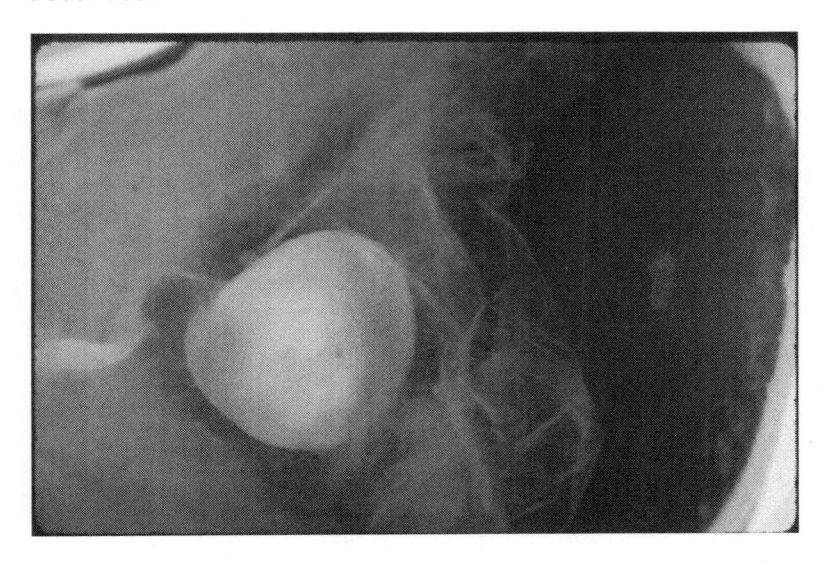

Dislocation of the lens in the eye.

About 1 in 5,000 people worldwide have been diagnosed with Marfan syndrome, which affects men and women equally. Due to difficulties in diagnosing mild Marfan syndrome, the condition might be under diagnosed, which means the actual figures might be much higher. It's a very common disorder; some research estimates that the number of people in the U.S. affected by MFS or similar connective-tissue disorders is about 200,000.

Sudden death due to undiagnosed MFS is relatively uncommon, but it does happen. American volleyball player Flo Hyman died suddenly in 1986 from a ruptured aorta caused by undiagnosed MFS. She was arguably the best American volleyball player to have lived. Dr. Victor Rosen, the pathologist who performed the autopsy, told the magazine Sports Illustrated *"There was no fat on her. She had tremendous muscle development. She had what we call a time-bomb lesion. Only no ticking is heard."*

College and professional sports teams now screen for Marfan syndrome and other height-connected pathologies like gigantism. This screening ended the career of Louisville basketball player Clarence Holloway in 2008 when he was diagnosed with MFS (Sports Illustrated).

Medical advances mean that most people with MFS can live normal, active lives. Lifestyle adaptations, such as avoidance of strenuous exercise and contact sports, are often necessary to reduce the risk of aortic dissection (tearing of the walls of the aorta). MFS patients are about 250 times more likely to suffer an aortic dissection than members of the general population.

If you or a loved one has MFS, this book will guide you through the condition and its treatment options. MFS is a difficult disorder to diagnose – even for medical professionals – and almost impossible to self-diagnose. In addition, MFS can be a life-threatening disorder that requires careful monitoring by medical professionals. This book should be used as a complement to medical care and should not be used to diagnose or treat MFS.

In the next chapter, we briefly cover the genetics behind Marfan syndrome, including how the disorder is inherited and which genes are responsible for the syndrome. Chapter 3 gives you information about signs and symptoms of MFS including the most common manifestations of the condition. In chapter 4, we take a look at how the condition is diagnosed and what you can expect when you visit the doctor for a diagnosis. Chapter 5 covers treatment options. Treatment is very individual and depends on what signs and symptoms you have. A lot of the "treatment" isn't treatment at all, but rather careful monitoring over your life for conditions like aortic dilation. Next is a short, but important chapter containing some information about what to do if you or your partner have MFS and are thinking about having children. After a listing of resources for MFS, we then highlight some other conditions which are similar to MFS. When you visit the doctor for an MFS diagnosis, it's often a "diagnosis of exclusion" which means that your physician will consider many other disorders and syndromes that involve the connective tissue. This section lists many of the connective tissue disorders with symptoms that overlap with Marfan syndrome.

We hope you find this book a useful tool in your journey with Marfan syndrome.

The Genetics of Marfan Syndrome

Marfan syndrome tends to run in families. It can be inherited from either parent or may be the result of a new mutation in about a quarter of cases. A new mutation means that you are the first person in your family to have the mutation.

Gene mutations that are passed from one of your parents are called hereditary mutations or germline mutations. The word "germline" is used because egg and sperm cells are also called germ cells.

It's also possible for a mutation to occur in either an egg or a sperm. In other words, a parent doesn't have the mutations but one of their germ cells does. These mutations are known as "de novo" mutations; de novo means "new". A third type of mutation is called an acquired or somatic mutation. These types of mutations can occur if a mistake is made when the DNA copies itself during development. Acquired mutations are not passed on to the next generation. However, all cases of MFS are either hereditary mutations (75%) or new mutations (25%), so if you have MFS you have a high risk (50%) of having children with the condition.

The only way to find out which type of MFS you have (hereditary or new) is to undergo genetic testing for both you and your first-degree relatives. First degree relatives are close family members: parents, siblings and your children.

Pattern of Inheritance

Marfan syndrome has an autosomal dominant pattern of inheritance. Autosomal dominant means that you only have to get the gene from one parent to be affected with the disease. Each MFS patient usually only has one parent who is affected, although it is possible for both parents to have MFS.

Autosomal dominant

Figure: Autosomal dominant inheritance pattern showing affected father and unaffected mother with four children: affected, unaffected, unaffected, affected. U.S. National Library of Medicine

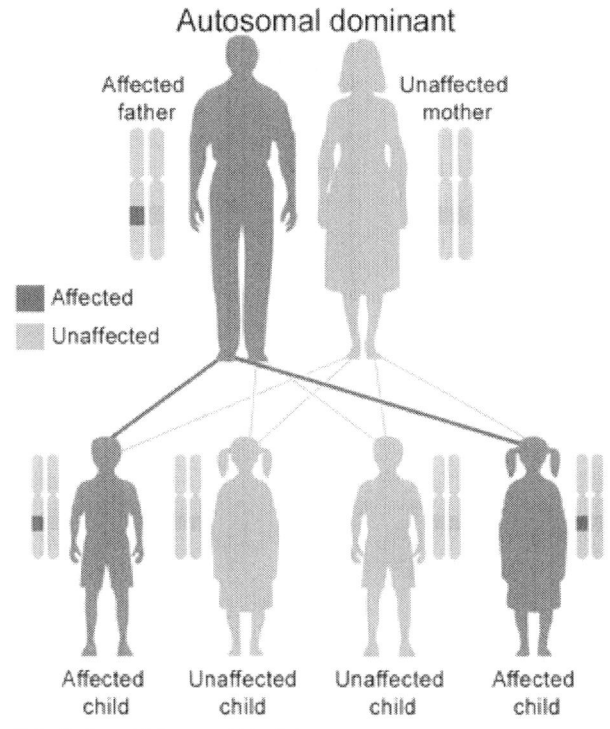

If a person with MFS chooses to have children, they have a 50 percent chance (1 in 2) of having a child with Marfan syndrome. If you have one child with Marfan syndrome, that fact does not affect whether a second child has MFS; each child has a 50% chance of acquiring the condition.

You have two copies of the FBN1 gene, but you only need to get one copy of a mutation in FNB1 to get the syndrome.

By 1998, 137 *FBN1* mutations had been discovered in patients with Marfan syndrome. These mutations are found throughout the *FBN1* gene (CHEN). Most mutations are one of three types:

1. **Missense mutations**. A missense mutation is when a single base pair changes. A base pair is made up of two chemical bases which are bonded to each other forming a "rung of the DNA ladder" (NIH). This change causes the substitution of a different amino acid (building blocks of proteins) in the resulting protein.

Missense mutation

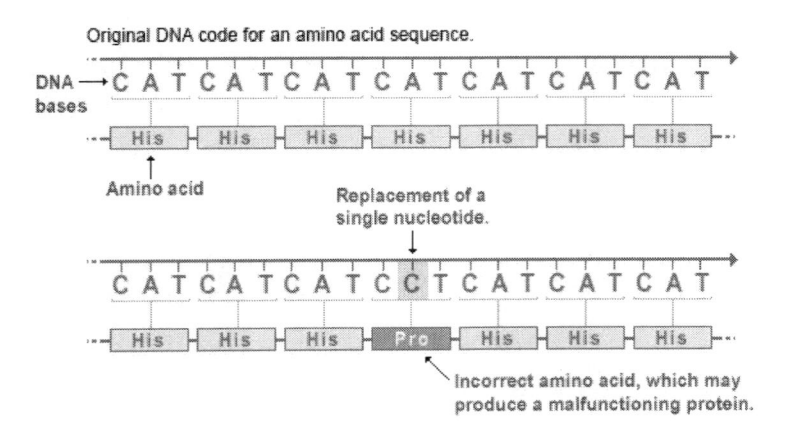

U.S. National Library of Medicine

2. **Small in-frame deletions**. In-frame deletions are where a part of the gene is deleted. Large deletions are normally lethal, but small

deletions can cause a myriad of conditions, including MFS.

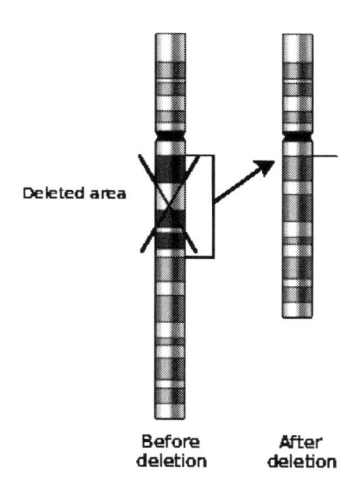

Before deletion / **After deletion** (Deleted area)

3. **Insertion mutations**, which change one peptide (a chain of amino acids) of around 3000 amino acids.

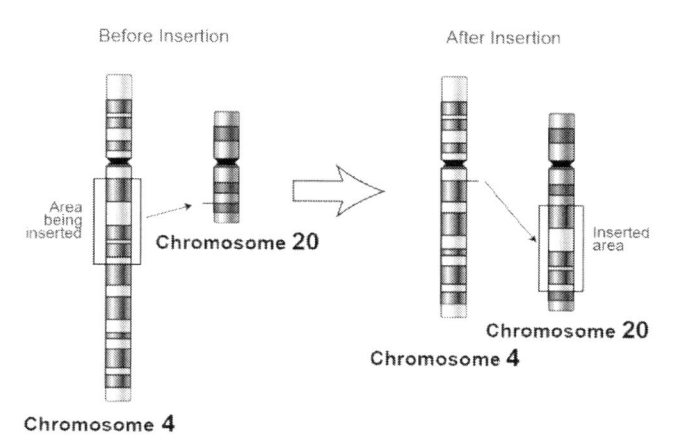

All of these three mutations to the FBN1 gene result in a mutant fibrillin-1 protein.

The FBN1 Gene ("fibrillin-1")

The FBN1 gene gives instructions for making fibrillin-1, a large protein that is transported out of your body's cells into an area called the extracellular matrix. The extracellular matrix is an elaborate network of proteins and molecules that fills the spaces in between the cells. Fibrillin-1's role is to bind to other molecules and proteins to form microfibrils, which turn into elastic fibers that allow the blood vessels, skin, and ligaments to stretch.

Microfibrils also give support to many other tissues in the body, including the lenses of your eyes, your muscles and your nerves. A FBN1 Mutation can lead to a decrease in the amount of fibrillin-1, which leads to fewer microfibrils being formed. One of the functions of microfibrils is to store transforming growth factor beta (TGF-β). With fewer microfibrils available to store the growth factor, an excess is released into the body, leading to taller stature and longer limbs and fingers. Additionally, the elasticity in tissues is decreased because of the lack of microfibrils. This leads to overgrowth and instability of tissue.

According to the National Institutes of Health, there are over 1,000 mutations of FBN1 that have been identified by researchers to date. Most of the FBN1 mutations involve a change to a single amino acid in the fibrillin-1 protein. The remainder of the FBN1 mutations results in a malfunctioning fibrillin-1 protein. The mutations may:

- Reduce the amount of fibrillin-1 produced by the cell.
- Alter the structure or stability of fibrillin-1.
- Impair the transport of fibrillin-1 out of the cell.

Genetic Maps

Geneticists use genetic maps to describe where genes are found on a chromosome. One type of map is called a cytogenetic location, which refers to where a particular band of a lab-stained chromosome lies. The FBN1 gene has a Cytogenetic Location of 15q21.1.

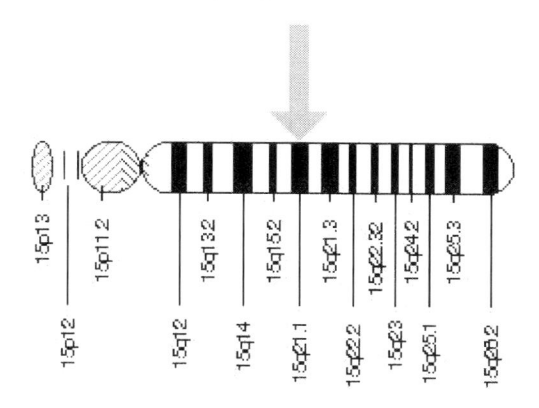

The cytogenetic location 15q21.1 tells us that the *FBN1* gene is located on the long (q) arm of chromosome 15 at position 21.1.

More precisely, the *FBN1* gene is located from base pair 48,408,305 to base pair 48,645,787 on chromosome 15.

Genetic Testing

If the genetic test is positive for a mutation of FBN1, this can confirm a suspected diagnosis of MFS. However, a negative result does not mean you do not have MFS. If you have clinical signs of MFS, the mutation is detected about 90% of the time. If you do not have clinical symptoms, you have about a 40% chance that you will not have a mutation identified. You may also have a *TGFβR2 mutation or a TGFβR1* mutation instead, which requires further genetic testing to find.

Genetic testing can identify exactly which mutation is present in the FBN1 gene and it can also track the gene through any particular family. However, sequencing genes to find these mutations is a very expensive, time-consuming and tedious undertaking. It's possible to have both false-positive and false-negative results. At the time of writing, best estimates put false-negatives at about 5% to 10%. In other words, the test is around 90-95% accurate. The cost is about $1400 to $2000 for initial mutation identification. If you need further tests (for example, to identify a deletion instead of a mutation), the cost will go up. Once the mutation is know, costs to test other family members are typically much lower, in the range of $240-$400 per patient.

Several other conditions are similar to MFS, and all are genetic conditions. If you do not have an FBN1 mutation, it's possible that you might have another genetic disorder.

Beals Syndrome

Signs and Symptoms: Mitral valve prolapse; skeletal findings.

Genes affected: FBN2

Vascular Ehlers-Danlos Syndrome

Signs and Symptoms: Skin and skeletal findings; aortic aneurysm/tear (selected types only).

Genes affected: COL3A1.

Familial Thoracic Aortic Aneurysm and Dissection

Signs and Symptoms: Aortic enlargement/tear; variable skeletal findings.

Genes affected: ACTA2, MYH11, MYLK, PRKG1 and, sometimes, FBN1.

Homocystinuria

Signs and Symptoms: Mitral valve prolapse; eye lens dislocation; skin and skeletal findings.

Genes affected: *CBS, MTHFR, MTR, MTRR,* and *MMADHC and others.*

Loeys-Dietz Syndrome

Signs and Symptoms: Aortic aneurysm/tear; skin and skeletal findings; arteries that twist and wind.

Genes affected: TGFBR1, TGFBR2.

Loeys-Dietz syndrome is a very severe syndrome that requires more aggressive monitoring and treatment than MFS.

Ectopia Lentis Syndrome

Signs and Symptoms: Eye lens dislocation; skeletal findings.

Genes affected: ADAMTS4L, FBN1.

MASS Phenotype

Signs and Symptoms: Mitral valve prolapse; myopia; borderline aortic enlargement; skin and skeletal findings.

Genes affected: sometimes FBN1, otherwise unknown.

Shprintzen-Goldberg Syndrome

Aortic enlargement; skin and skeletal findings.

Genes affected: SKI and, rarely, FBN1.

Stickler Syndrome

Signs and Symptoms: Eye features; some skeletal findings.

Genes affected: COL2A1, COL11A1, COL11A2, COL9A1, COL9A2.

If you are interested in genetic testing, ask your physician for a referral to a genetic counselor. At the time of writing, there are more than 500 genetic testing laboratories in the US. The procedure requires blood samples from the patients who require the testing. Sometimes, your insurance may pay for genetic testing but you may have to pay out-of-pocket.

Genetic testing is regulated by the federal government. For more information on the regulations, visit www.genome.gov. For a list of laboratories that perform genetic testing, visit genetests.org and select the Laboratory Directory link.

Signs and Symptoms

The specific signs or symptoms of Marfan syndrome vary from person to person. One person might have many symptoms while another person may have no signs or symptoms at all. It can be hard to make a diagnosis of Marfan syndrome in the very early childhood years, as it can take some time for symptoms to show. If MFS is diagnosed in infancy, the syndrome tends to take a more severe course than if it is diagnosed later in life. Most MFS patients are diagnosed before the age of 10 although some people are not diagnosed until they reach adulthood or are never diagnosed at all until it's too late (like Flo

Hyman). If diagnosed in an infant, the prognosis is poor; there are very few studies which address this issue so it's extremely hard to come to any conclusions about what you can expect if your infant is diagnosed with MFS. One study (Morse) of 54 infants with MFS showed that the vast majority (between 83 and 94 percent) had serious heart problems or congenital contractures (a condition where the muscles are shortened or contracted). Heart problems tended to worsen and often led to death or severe disability.

Signs and symptoms are wide and varied, overlapping with many other genetic disorders. Typically, people with Marfan syndrome are very tall and slender with extremely long arms and legs. Abnormal curvature of the spine or chest wall is also very common, as are loose joints and ligaments. About 90% of people with Marfan syndrome have issues with the heart and blood vessels. People with Marfan syndrome commonly have some of these signs and symptoms:

General Appearance

In general, MFS patients tend to have a very tall and thin frame compared to members of their family. Arms, legs, fingers and toes may look very long when compared with the trunk of the body. Faces tend to be long and narrow as well. In infants, the eyes may be deep set and they may look older than siblings of around the same age. MFS patients may have crowded teeth and a highly arched palate (the roof of the mouth). Overbites, where the lower jaw recedes, are also common. In general, MFS patients also have abnormally flexible joints.

Pectus excavatum or pectus carinatum

Pectus excavatum is a chest that sinks in and pectus carinatum is a chest that sticks out. Severe pectus excavatum can compromise how your heart and lungs work.

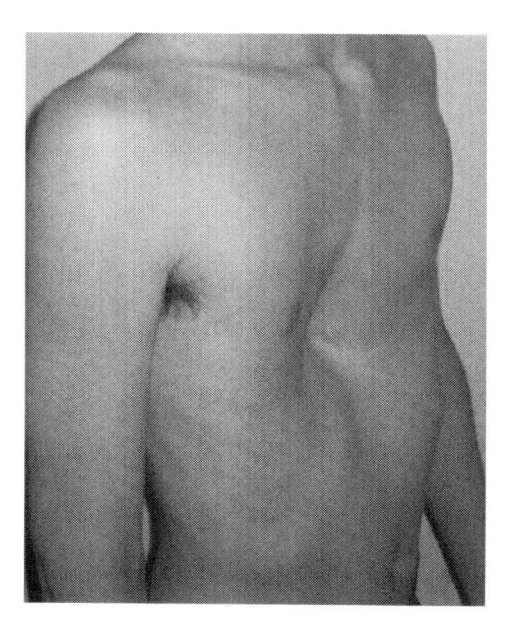

Pectus excavatum

Stretch marks not caused by pregnancy or weight loss.

Stretch marks on the skin are common in Marfan syndrome and usually appear on the lower back, buttocks, shoulders, breasts, thighs, and abdomen. Although you might feel embarrassed by their presence, they are not any cause for concern and there is no treatment necessary for them.

Scoliosis

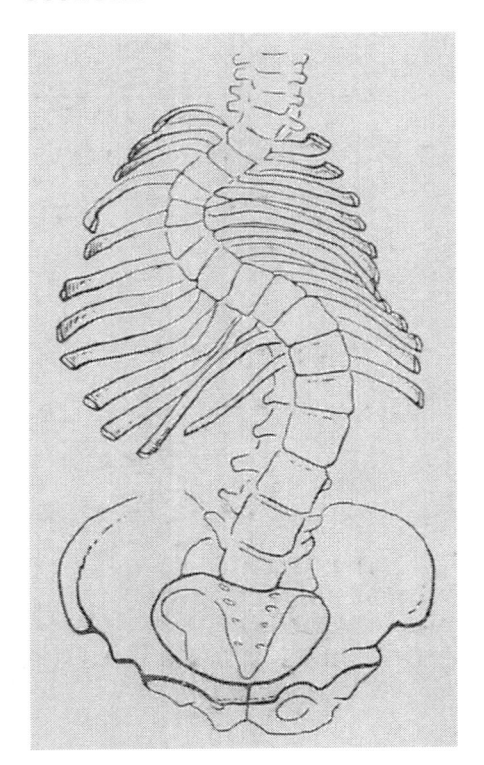

Scoliosis is a spine that curves to the left or right, usually in a spiral or S-shape. Scoliosis usually affects the upper part of the spine. It's caused because the ligaments that normally hold the spine straight are loose. If a child with MFS hasn't developed scoliosis by the beginning of middle school, there is a very low risk of it happening later in life.

Kyphosis (Hunched back)

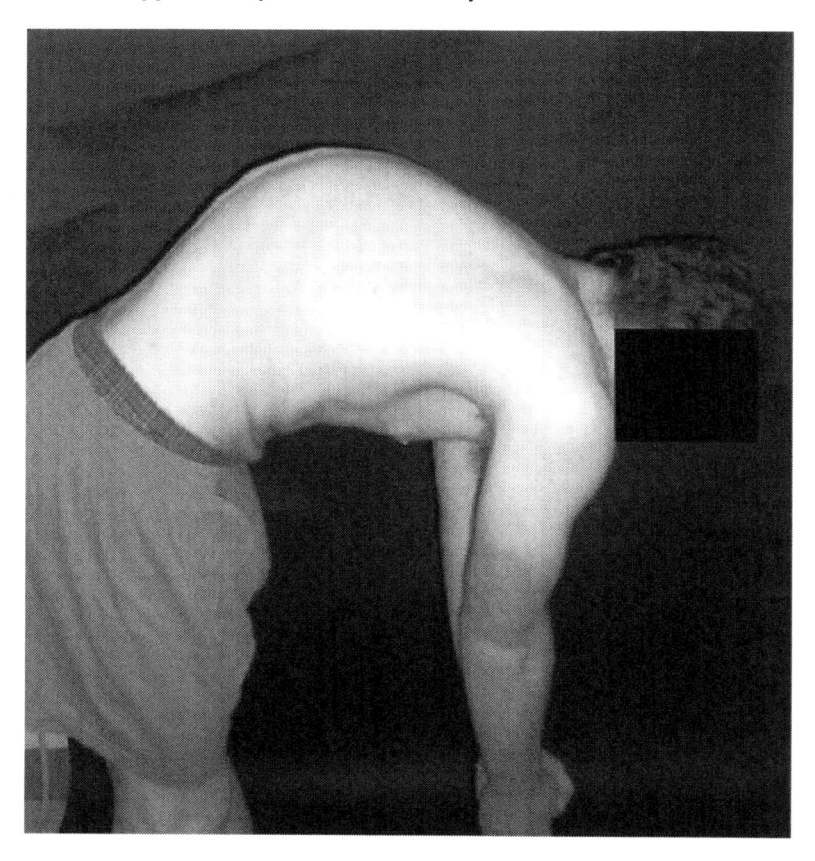

The normal back, when viewed from the side, has a slight curve of between 20 and 45 degrees. Any more than 45 degrees is called kyphosis. Although kyphosis is usually seen in the upper spine, MFS patients can have the condition in the upper spine or in the lower spine.

Feet problems

People with MFS have long and slender feet. Weakened ligaments in the feet can lead to a variety of signs and conditions including:

- Flat feet
- Hammer or claw toes
- Calluses caused by a large amount of pressure on one area of the foot
- Bunions (excessive bone growth near the base of the big toes)
- Turned ankles

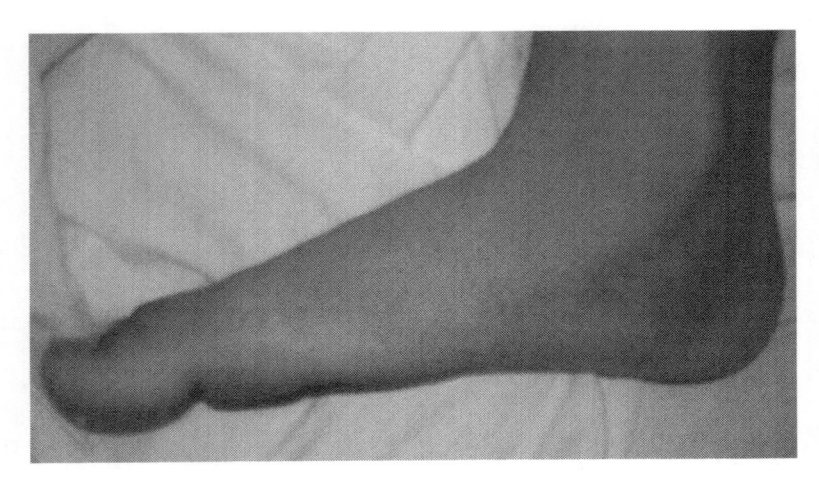

Picture on previous page: A flat foot

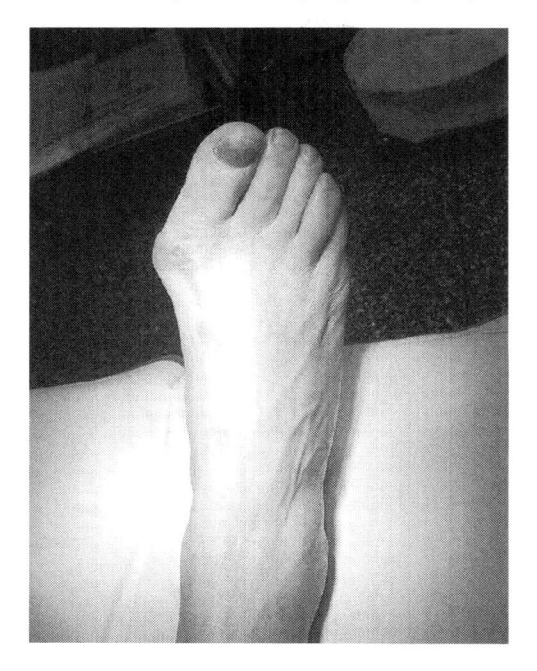

Above: A bunion

Eye problems

MFS patients can suffer from severe nearsightedness (myopia), astigmatism (blurred vision), amblyopia (lazy eye) or strabismus (where your two eyes do not focus on an object at the same time). In amblyopia, vision in one eye deteriorates while with strabismus, the eye is out of alignment but you have normal vision. Many other problems can affect you if you have MFS, including a flattened or enlarged cornea (the outer part of the eye), difficulty with pupil dilation (sometimes seen with eye exams when the ophthalmologist attempts to dilate your eyes), and enophthalmos (sunken in eyeballs). About 35 percent of MFS patients will develop glaucoma, a condition caused by increased pressure in the eye. You are also at a higher risk for a dislocated lens, retinal detachment or early cataracts.

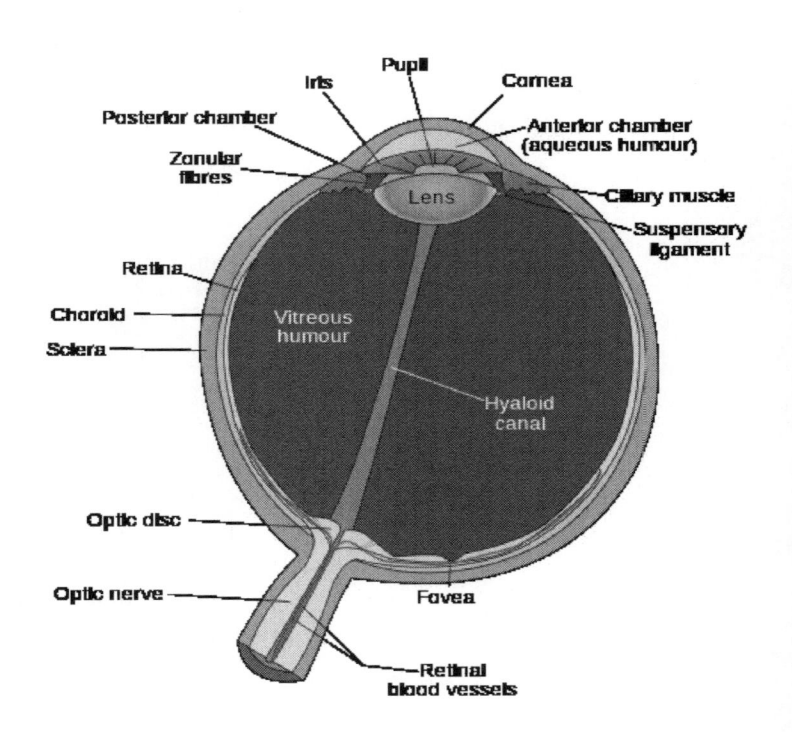

Dislocated Lens

The lens is a transparent structure located behind the iris that helps to focus on objects. The lens may dislocate because the zonule of Zinn (the connective tissue that holds the lenses in place) is weak. Symptoms may be mild to severe and can include blurry vision, nearsightedness and fluctuating vision. An ophthalmologist can determine if you have a dislocated lens by conducting a slit-lamp eye examination with your eyes fully dilated. Although dislocated lenses are rare in the general population, about 60 percent of MFS patients have the condition.

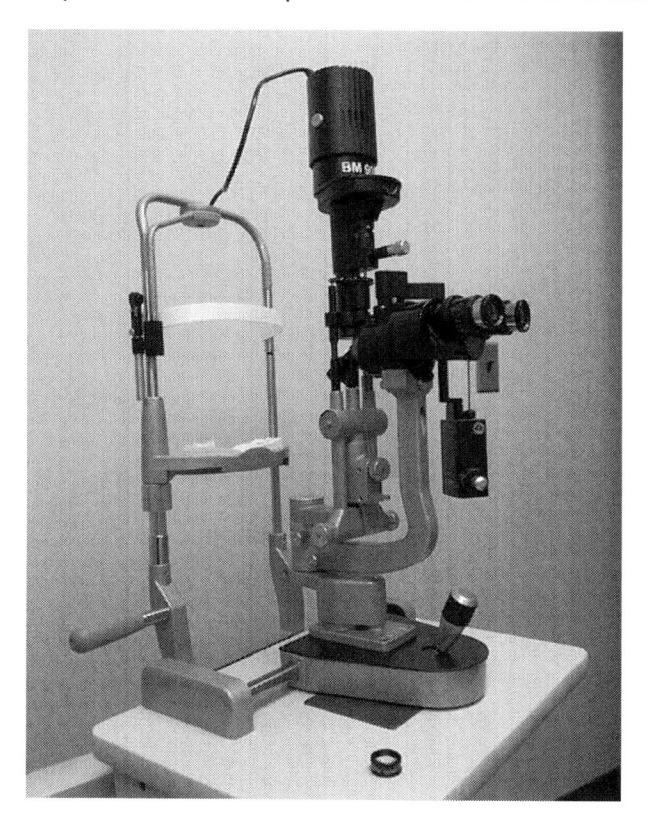

A slit lamp machine shines a bright light into the eye

Detached retina

The retina is the light-sensitive membrane in the back of your eye. A detached retina can cause:

- Floaters
- Blurred vision
- Flashing lights
- A gray curtain across your field of vision.

If you suspect you may have retinal detachment, see an eye doctor immediately. The sooner the condition is treated (within about 24 hours of detachment), the lower the chance of blindness. A detached retina can be detected with a slit lamp exam.

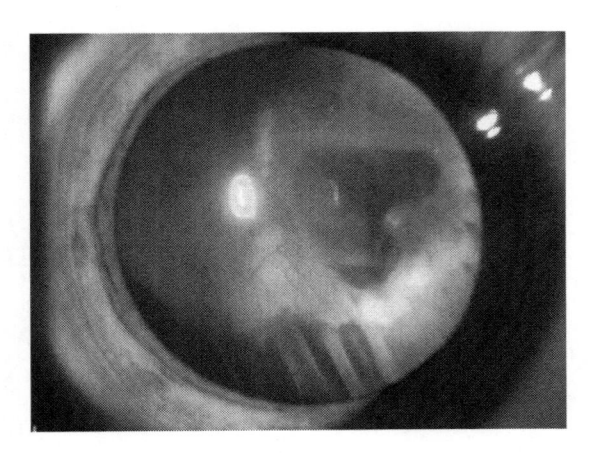

A detached retina as shown on a slit lamp exam

Early Cataracts

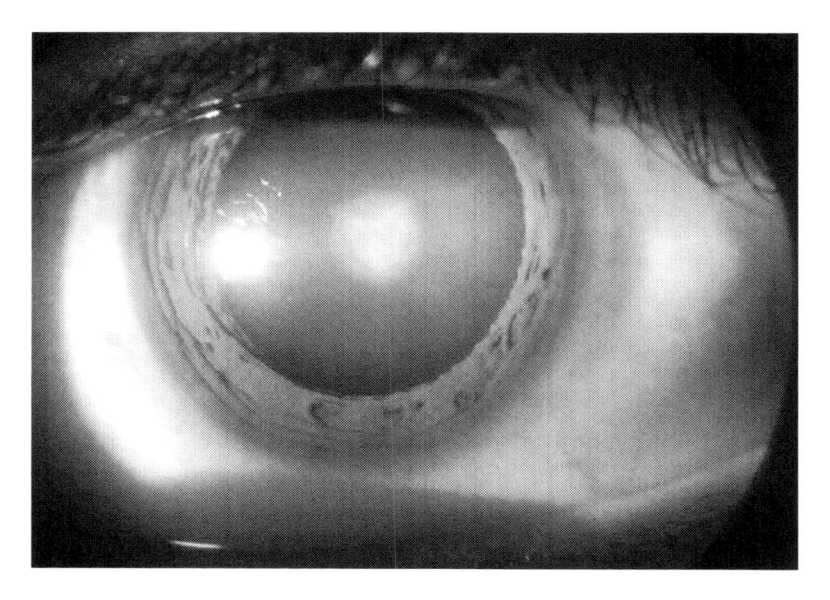

A cataract is a clouding of the lens of the eye. Although cataracts usually affect the general population after the age of 60, MFS patients can get cataracts earlier. Sometimes, this can happen before the age of 40.

Dural Ecstasia

More than 60 percent of MFS patients have an enlarged dura (the dura is a membrane that surrounds the brain and spinal cord). For the vast majority of patients, dural ecstasia occurs in the lowest part of the spine, where the pressure is greatest from standing. This can cause pain in the head, back or abdomen although some patients may not experience any symptoms at all. Dural ecstasia can thin the vertebrae in your spine. Although this generally does not cause problems, it can have implications if you need surgery on your spine. In extreme cases surgery may be needed to repair the dura.

Heart Problems

About 90 percent of people with Marfan syndrome have problems with their heart or blood vessels. If the aortic vessels are affected, surgery may be necessary to replace the aorta (a procedure called aortic root replacement). Complications that affect the aorta are the primary cause of death in people with MFS.

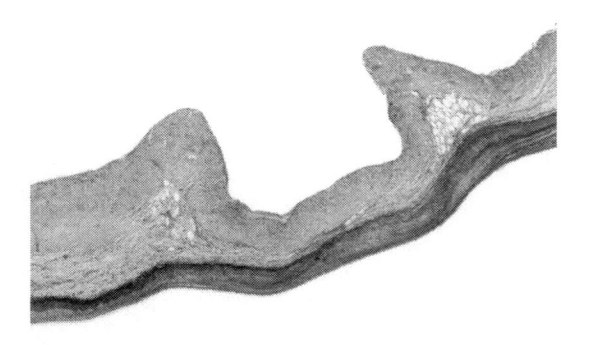

Micrograph demonstrating myxomatous degeneration (weakening of the connective tissue) of the aortic valve.

Aortic Dissection

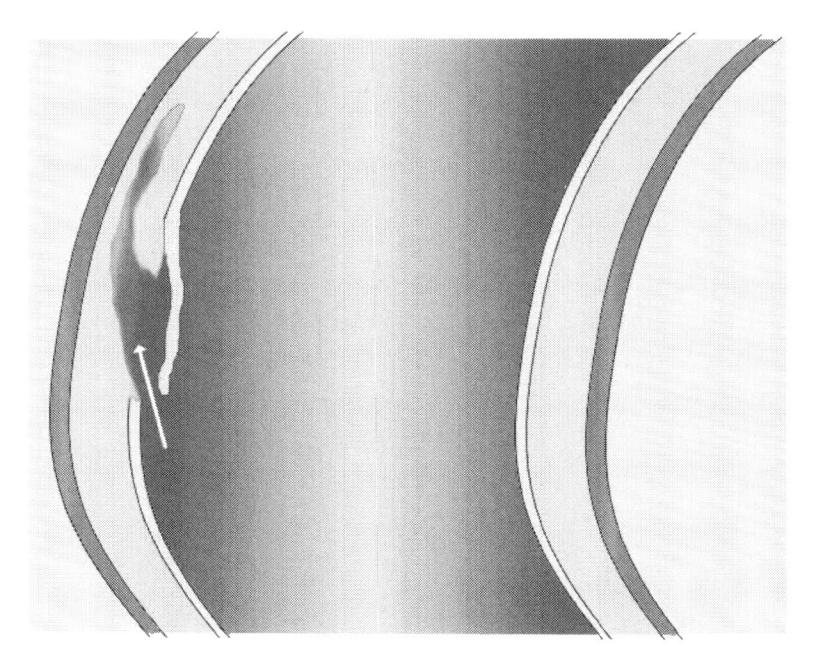

The aorta is made up of three layers, the *intima*, the *media*, and the *adventitia*. The intima is in direct contact with the blood inside the vessel, and mainly consists of a layer of endothelial cells (the thin layer of cells that lines the interior surface of blood vessels and lymphatic vessels) on a basement membrane; the media contains connective and muscle tissue, and the vessel is protected on the outside by the adventitia, comprising connective tissue.

In an aortic dissection, blood penetrates the *intima* and enters the *media* layer. The high pressure rips the tissue of the *media* apart along the laminated plane splitting the inner 2/3 and the outer 1/3 of the media apart.

Aortic dissection usually causes severe pain in the chest, stomach or back which is sometimes described as a ripping or tearing sensation.

There are two types of aortic dissection: dissection of the ascending aorta (the part closest to the heart) and dissection of the descending aorta (the part that goes down into the chest cavity and below the waist). Dissections of the ascending aorta are more common with MFS and they are a life-threatening medical emergency. In most cases, dissections of the descending aorta can be managed with medication and careful monitoring. Some cases may require surgery.

Aortic dissection can lead to a rupture and is a medical emergency. It can result in:

- Lethal hemorrhage, a condition where the patient bleeds too much.

- Acute aortic valvular insufficiency, a condition that results in a sudden increase of blood to the left ventricle of the heart. The ventricle is unable to keep up with the sudden influx of blood. This is a medical emergency which requires immediate surgery for aortic valve replacement.

If you think you have an aortic dissection, call 911 immediately. Lay down if you can, and try to remain calm; panic causes your heart to beat faster, putting more pressure on your aorta.

"I had an aortic dissection in 2008. Unfortunately, because of my location (I live near a mountain town), it took a couple of hours to get to a trauma center. I tried my best to remain calm and not panic, and I laid down. The doctor told me those actions (or inactions) may have saved my life as it slowed the dissection. It wasn't until several hours later, when I sat up suddenly, that the dissection reached an emergency state." Paul, Drake, Colorado.

Emergency personnel may not think of aortic dissection initially, unless you inform them you have MFS. As you may not be able to communicate well in an emergency situation, you should consider wearing a Medic-Alert bracelet.

According to the Cleveland Clinic, about 40 percent of MFS patients will die immediately with an aortic dissection and for every hour that follows, the risk of death is between 1 and 3 percent. If surgery is performed *before* an aortic dissection occurs (in other words, if you have preventative surgery), there is a 98 percent survival rate.

Mitral valve prolapse (MVP)

Mitral valve prolapse is a "floppy" mitral valve that doesn't close properly. MVP is a very common heart abnormality; according to the National Institutes of Health, about 3% of people in the general population have it. Many (but not all) Marfan patients have mitral valve prolapse (Weyman). It may not cause symptoms, but if the MVP is causing blood to flow back into the left atrium, it may cause palpitations, irregular heartbeats (arrhythmias) and shortness of breath. The extent of the MVP is measured by how displaced the leaflets (the flaps) are. A displacement of over 2mm is normally cause for concern, as this may lead to increased leaflet thickness, valve-related complications, or mitral insufficiency (Weyman).

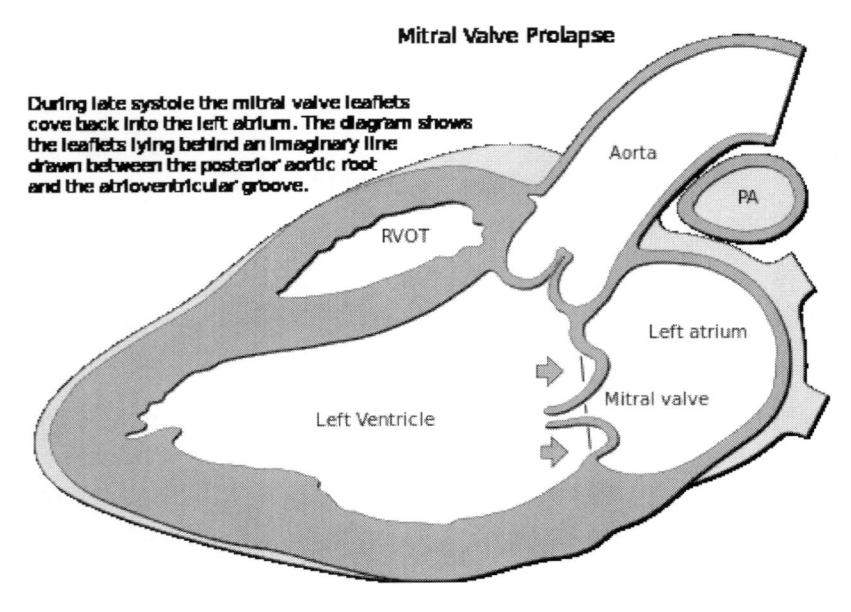

Mitral Valve Prolapse

During late systole the mitral valve leaflets cove back into the left atrium. The diagram shows the leaflets lying behind an imaginary line drawn between the posterior aortic root and the atrioventricular groove.

Aorta
PA
RVOT
Left atrium
Mitral valve
Left Ventricle

Mitral insufficiency

Mitral insufficiency (also called mitral valve regurgitation) is a disorder where the mitral valve does not close properly. The mitral valve separates the upper and lower chambers of the heart. This can lead to congestive heart failure or severe arrhythmias (problems with your heart's rhythm) and is the most common cause of death in children with Marfan syndrome. Treatment depends on how severe your signs and symptoms are. If you have mild mitral insufficiency, no treatment may be necessary. However, heart surgery to repair the valve may be needed if your signs and symptoms are severe.

Pericardial tamponade

Pericardial tamponade is where fluid collects in the sac surrounding the heart. This prevents the heart ventricles from expanding fully and your body may not receive enough blood. Symptoms include anxiety, chest pain, difficulty breathing, palpitations, rapid breathing, fainting or a pale, gray, or blue skin. The condition can be diagnosed with an echocardiogram. Pericardial tamponade is a medical emergency. If you receive prompt treatment, the prognosis is usually good. Treatment may involve giving fluids to maintain blood pressure, followed by surgery (called pericardiocentesis).

Bacterial endocarditis

Bacterial endocarditis is a condition where bacteria in the bloodstream enter an inner portion of the heart. It can occur after surgeries and procedures. If left untreated, endocarditis can destroy your heart valves. It can be treated with antibiotics, although some cases may require surgery.

Aortic dilation

Aortic dilation is where the aorta becomes enlarged. An aorta that is severely enlarged carries a higher risk for rupturing or tearing. For adults, you'll often hear the aorta measured in millimeters (mm). Anything over 40mm starts to be cause for concern. In children, a *z-score* is usually used to take into account age, height and weight. Z-scores are used in statistics to measure how far from the mean (the average) a certain score is. In pediatric cardiology, z-scores can tell a physician how far a patient's aorta size is from what would be expected in the "average" person of that age, height and weight (Chubb). Z-scores are used because the size of the aorta changes with age and what's more important is the size of the aorta relative to the size of the patient. There are many z-score calculators online that you can use for calculating a pediatric z-score (search for "z score aortic root"). This condition can be treated with surgery (see the next chapter for more information on surgery for aortic dilation).

Aneurysms

If you have MFS, you are at a higher risk for an aneurysm. Preventative screening is usually recommended.

An aneurysm (AN-u-rism) is a balloon-like bulge in an artery. The arteries are oxygen-rich blood vessels, carrying oxygen to different parts of your body. Arteries have thick walls to resist typical blood pressure level. These arteries may be weaker in MFS patients. The force of blood pushing against the weakened or injured walls can result in an aneurysm.

Most aneurysms in MFS occur inside the aorta, the leading artery that carries oxygen-rich blood from your heart. The aorta goes through the chest and abdomen.

An aneurysm is a medical emergency that can cause dangerous bleeding inside the body, including a dissection or rupture.

Figure A on the following page shows a normal aorta. Figure B shows a thoracic aortic aneurysm (which is located behind the heart). Figure C shows an abdominal aortic aneurysm located below the arteries that supply blood to the kidneys.

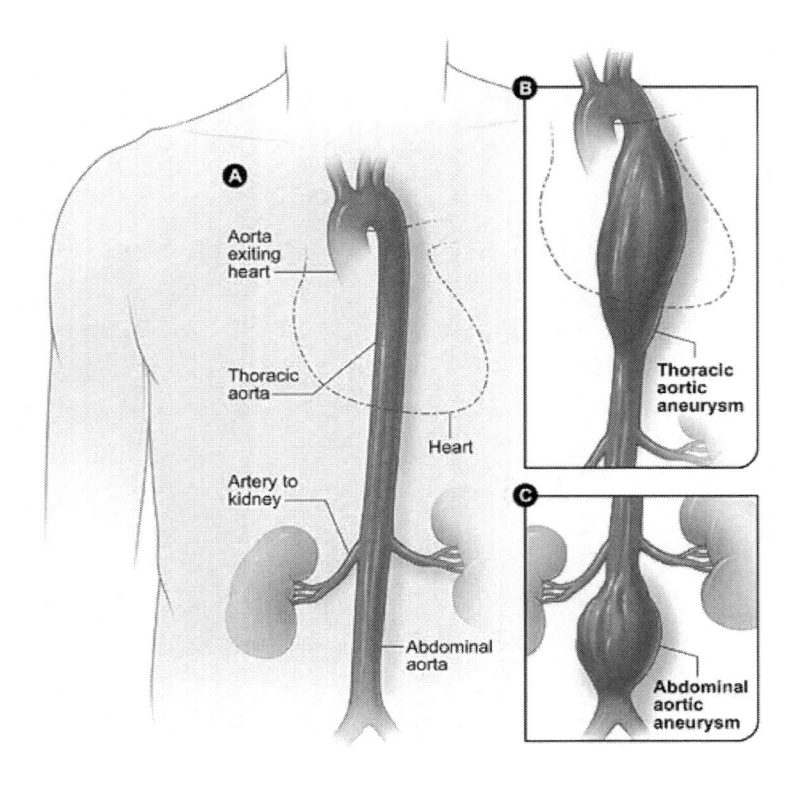

Thoracic aortic aneurysm (TAA)

An aneurysm that occurs in the chest part of the aorta is known as a thoracic aortic aneurysm. Aortic aneurysms can lead to aortic dissection (a tear in the inner wall of the aorta). TAAs are typically are repaired with surgery. Early detection and intervention are critical because aneurysms and dissections can lead to a rupture and massive internal bleeding. Symptoms of an aortic aneurysm can include:

- Pain in your chest, back or neck.
- Severe chest/back pain that feels like ripping or tearing. The pain may move around.
- Swelling in your head, neck and arms.
- Trouble breathing, coughing or wheezing.
- Coughing up blood.
- Pale skin.
- Faint pulse.
- Numbness and tingling.
- Paralysis.
- A fear of impending death.

About 20 percent of people with thoracic aortic aneurysm have a familial history, called familial thoracic aortic aneurysm and dissection (FTAAD). In other words, it runs in the family. The condition does not always cause symptoms, which is why preventative screening is a must.

Abdominal aortic aneurysms (AAAs)

Most abdominal aortic aneurysms (AAAs) happen slowly but surely. They generally do not trigger signs or signs until they rupture. If you have an AAA, your physician could feel a throbbing mass when checking your abdomen.

When signs or symptoms are present, you could have:
- A throbbing sensation in the abdomen.
- Deep pain in your back or your abdomen.
- Steady, gnawing pain within your abdomen that lasts for hours or days.

If an AAA ruptures, signs or symptoms might include:
- Sudden, severe pain inside your abdomen and back.
- Nausea (feeling ill in your stomach) and vomiting.
- Constipation and difficulties with urination.
- Clammy, sweaty skin.
- Light-headedness; along with a rapid heart rate when standing up.

Internal bleeding from a ruptured aorta can send you into shock. If you suspect you have an aneurysm or dissection, this can be life-threatening and requires prompt medical treatment.

Surgery, such as a Bentall procedure or valve-sparing surgery, is most effective *before* a dissection has happened. A Bentall procedure involves composite graft replacement of the aortic valve, aortic root and ascending aorta, with re-implantation of the coronary arteries into the graft.

Brain Aneurysms

A brain aneurysm is an abnormal bulge or "ballooning" in the wall of an artery in the brain. They are sometimes called berry aneurysms because they are often the size of a small berry. Most brain aneurysms produce no symptoms until they become large, begin to leak blood, or burst. There is some debate about the risks for brain aneurysms in Marfan syndrome patients. Some authors (including Conway) conclude that the risks are about the same as in the general population. Other authors suggest an increased risk (Schievink).

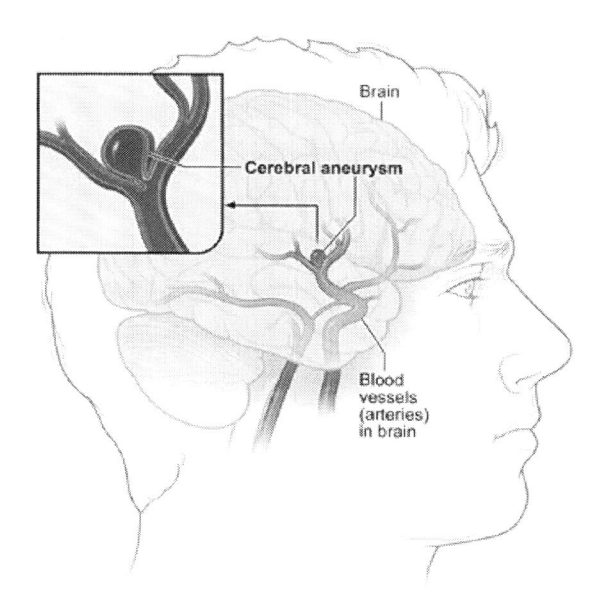

If a brain aneurysm presses on nerves in your brain, it can cause signs and symptoms. These can include

- A droopy eyelid.
- Double vision or other changes in vision.
- Pain above or behind the eye.
- A dilated pupil.
- Numbness or weakness on one side of the face or body.

Treatment depends on the size and location of the aneurysm, whether it is infected, and whether it has burst. If a brain aneurysm bursts, symptoms can include a sudden, severe headache, nausea and vomiting, stiff neck, loss of consciousness, and signs of a stroke. Any of these symptoms requires immediate medical attention.

Restrictive Lung Disease

Over 70 percent of people with MFS also have restrictive lung disease. Restrictive lung disease restricts the expansion of the lungs and makes it difficult to take breaths, especially during exertion or increased activity. The main symptoms are coughing and shortness of breath. This is a very common condition in MFS patients; about 7 out of 10 MFS patients have restrictive lung disease. The cause could be muscle weakness or skeletal issues like pectus excavatum or scoliosis. According to Enid Neptune,

MD, an adult pulmonologist and developmental biologist at the Johns Hopkins School of Medicine, surgery, such as corrective surgery for pectus excavatum, may enable you to maintain your level of lung function or it may improve it. However, many surgeries have potential complications and may not improve lung function; you should discuss your surgical options and the reasons for any surgery with your physician.

Spontaneous Pneumothorax (Sudden Lung Collapse)

A pneumothorax is an abnormal collection of gas or air in the space between the lung and the chest wall that collapses the lung. The pain may resemble a heart attack and can be a medical emergency; if you suspect you have a pneumothorax, seek immediate medical attention. Spontaneous pneumothorax is one of the most common lung conditions in Marfan syndrome; MFS patients are several hundred times more likely to have spontaneous pneumothorax than the general population (Wood).

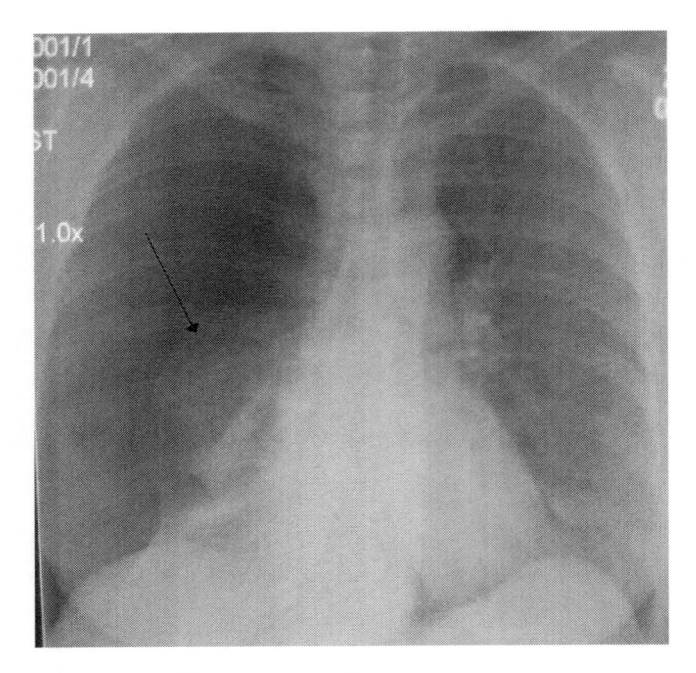

An X-ray of a pneumothorax

Emphysema

When the walls of the lungs are damaged, they cannot push all of the air out of the lungs. This condition, called emphysema, affects around 10 percent of MFS patients. Symptoms of emphysema include shortness of breath, coughing and wheezing.

Sleep apnea

Sleep apnea is a condition that interrupts your sleep. When your breathing pauses or becomes shallow, it can disrupt your deep sleep. This results in poor quality of sleep and tiredness. Symptoms include loud snoring or pauses in snoring (which may be noticed by your partner), a dry mouth and sore throat when you wake up, sleepiness during the day and morning headaches. Untreated sleep apnea in MFS patients can lead to stress in the aortic walls, which makes it very important to diagnose and treat the disorder.

These are some of the most common signs and symptoms of Marfan symptom. However, it is a connective tissue disorder, which means that technically it could affect *any* part of your body.

Diagnosis

Although genetic testing can help with a diagnosis of Marfan syndrome, it isn't used on its own for diagnostic purposes. One reason for this is that mutation detection isn't a perfect science and many other diseases can be associated with an FBN1 mutation or have Marfan-like symptoms and signs, including:

- Weill-Marchesani syndrome, another connective tissue disorder. An eye disorder called microspherophakia is associated with this syndrome.

Microspherophakia refers to a small, sphere-shaped lens.

- Stiff skin syndrome, which is characterized by very hard, thick skin covering most of the body.

- Acromicric dysplasia, a disorder associated with a very short stature, short limbs, stiff joints, and distinctive facial features.

- MASS syndrome, which causes abnormalities in several parts of the body, including the mitral valve, the aorta, the skeleton, and the skin.

- Shprintzen-Goldberg syndrome, which can cause premature fusion of some bones of the skull. This affects the shape of the head and face. Other features include long, slender fingers and toes and intellectual disability.

- Ehlers-Danlos Syndrome also affects the connective tissues, but unlike MFS, the joint and skin problems are due to issues with collagen, proteins that stabilize the connective tissue and give it elasticity.

MFS can usually be diagnosed without genetic testing. However, there is no single test that leads to a diagnosis of MFS. Your physician will reach a diagnosis by a combination of techniques including looking at your personal and family history, conducting a physical exam and requesting a number of specialized tests. It's recommended that you find a physician who is knowledgeable about the condition. As MFS is not a common disorder, not all doctors are familiar with the condition. Your best bet is to find a medical geneticist (a physician whose specialty is genetic disorders). If there is no medical geneticist in your area, a cardiologist (a heart doctor) would be the next best choice.

Before you visit the doctor, compile a complete personal and family history. The history should include all family members who have MFS and any family members who died from heart or vascular issues. You should also list all of your illnesses, conditions and hospitalizations and the reasons why you think you might have MFS.

The most recent set of criteria for diagnosing MFS is called the Ghent criteria, or Ghent Nosology (2010). A family history of MFS, dislocation of the lens in the eye, and an aortic root aneurysm (the aortic root is the part of the aorta that is closest to the heart) weighs heavily in this criteria. The Ghent criteria is broken up into two sections: major and minor criteria.

Major criteria include:

• An enlarged aorta (the main artery).

• A tear in the aorta.

- A dislocation of the lens of the eye (ectopia lentis).

- A family history of the syndrome.

- At least four skeletal problems, such as flat feet or a curved spine (scoliosis).

- Dural ecstasia, an enlargement of the lining that surrounds part of the spinal cord.

Minor criteria include:

- Short-sightedness (myopia).

- Unexplained stretch marks. Some MFS patients have stretch marks on the shoulders, back and thighs. These stretch marks may appear even though a patient hasn't lost weight or been pregnant.

- Loose joints.

- A long, thin face.

- A high, arched palate (roof of the mouth).

The "Thumb sign" can also be used to aid a diagnosis. The following image shows a normal thumb sign at the top and a MFS thumb sign at the bottom.

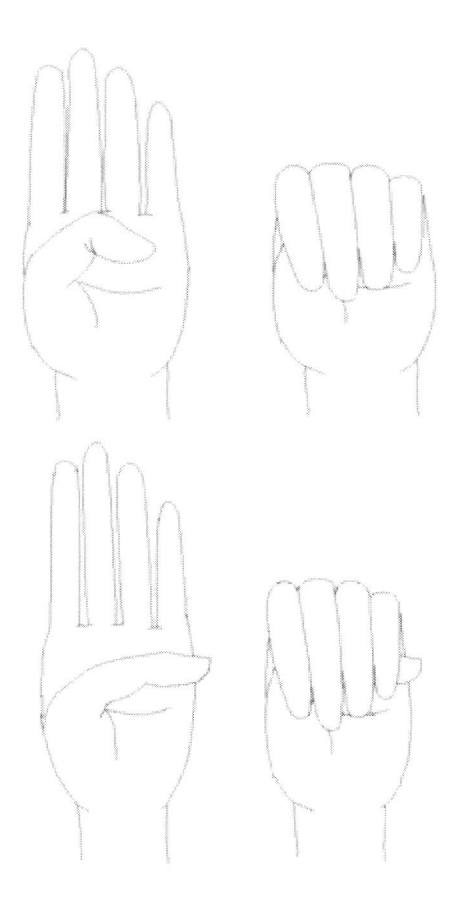

Your doctor may also look at you and your family's genetics when arriving at a diagnosis of MFS:

1. Genetic testing: Presence of an *FBN1* mutation known to cause MFS.

2. Family history: A first-degree relative (parent, child, or sibling) who meets

the diagnostic criteria. Family members have at least one organ system majorly affected and a second organ system affected to some degree.

3. Inheritance of an *FBN1* haplotype known to be associated with MFS in the family. A FBN1 haplotype is a group of alleles that are located close to each other on the FBN1 gene and tend to be inherited together.

If there is no familial history of MFS, the criteria changes a little, A person must have major involvement in two separate organ systems and involvement in a third organ system.

Because of the expense and unreliability of genetic testing, a diagnosis of MFS is mostly clinical and depends on the knowledge and expertise of your physician, who will look for several signs and symptoms to figure out what organ systems are involved (Chen). These include:

- Delayed developmental milestones like crawling, walking and grasping objects caused by loose ligaments in the hips, knees, ankles, foot arches, wrists and fingers.
- Heart murmurs or an irregular heartbeat.
- Indications of a tear in the inner wall of the aorta. Symptoms include an abrupt

onset of chest pain, faintness, pallor, and paralysis in the arms and legs.
- Signs and symptoms of dural ectasia (a widening or ballooning of the dural sac around the spinal cord). Symptoms include low back pain, burning or weakness in the legs and a headache. The vast majority of people with MFS have dural ecstasia (65-92%).
- Joint pain (adults).
- Shortness of breath, heart palpitations or pain in the sternum area caused by pectus excavatum (sunken in chest). Shortness of breath and chest pain can also be caused by a collection of air or gas in the space between the lungs and the chest that collapses the lung (spontaneous pneumothorax).
- A protruding chest (pectus carinatum) is also seen in MFS patients. However, pectus carinatum does not cause the heart and lung issues of a sunken in chest.
- Visual problems from a dislocated lens or detached retina. About half of MFS patients have a dislocated lens (ectopia lentis). Some other eyes problems are sometimes seen in MFS patients, including a flat cornea, early (under aged 50) cataracts and glaucoma, and nearsightedness.
- A very tall and thin frame, compared to other family members, along with

very long arms and legs which are disproportionately long compared to the body.
- Very long, spider-like fingers (arachnodactyly).
- Scoliosis (where the spine is curved from side to side), flat feet, hip deformations, crowded teeth, and highly arched palates (the roof of the mouth) are also seen in many MFS patients.

Diagnosis is sometimes more problematic in young children, because many of the physical features do not show up in early childhood. A positive DNA test or a family history of MFS can help your physician reach the right diagnosis. However, a negative DNA test does not always mean that a child does not have MFS. If there aren't enough physical signs of MFS, your doctor may recommend yearly evaluations for your child until they reach 18 years-old or until a diagnosis of MFS is made.

When you first meet your physician for a diagnosis, they will ask you about your personal and family histories to start the diagnostic process. You'll also have a physical examination, including an eye exam and an echocardiogram to look for possible heart problems. An echocardiogram uses sound waves to make a picture of the heart. Unlike x-rays, no radiation is involved. You doctor may also recommend transesophageal echocardiography (TEE) to get more detailed pictures of the heart. In TEE, a flexible tube with a probe at the tip is guides down your esophagus (the tube that leads from your mouth to your stomach).

If you have scoliosis or issues with your hip socket (a condition called protrusio acetabulae), you'll also need x-rays of these areas. An MRI of your pelvis may be necessary if your doctor suspects you have dural ecstasia (a widening or ballooning of the sac around the spinal cord).

MRI

An MRI is a safe, painless technique to produce detailed 3-D images of your body. Although the test is painless, many people feel claustrophobic during the test, as you'll lay on a stretcher in a tube for the procedure. The machine itself is extremely noisy (you'll hear loud, random banging sounds) and takes around 45 minutes to complete – during which time you'll have to lay completely still. You'll be given ear protection and a "panic button" so that you can alert the technician if you have difficulties during the test. If you have an issue with claustrophobia, you can ask your doctor to provide a mild sedative (like Valium) for the procedure.

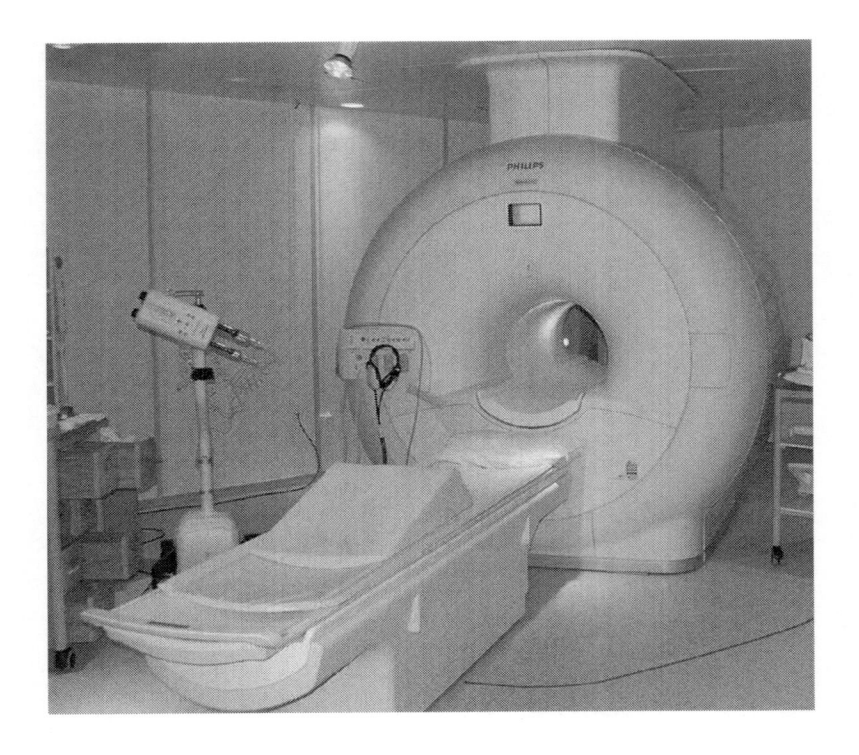

MRIs are extremely safe, and there are no known side effects from the imaging procedure itself. On the rare occasion the machine does cause harm, it's usually unrelated to the imaging itself. Make sure you tell the technician if you have any metal in your body. You'll be given a comprehensive questionnaire when you arrive for the test which will ask about potential objects that can cause issues – make sure you read it completely. Aneurysm clips and pacemakers are just two devices that could cause serious issues. In addition, some MRI accidents have happened because of:

1. Projectiles. The MRI is a giant magnet and on rare occasions, objects have been sucked into the magnetic field. In 2001, a child was killed when an oxygen canister was sucked into the machine.
2. Burns. Don't touch the walls of the MRI tunnel as it carries the risk of severe burns. If there is a risk of you coming into contact with the wall, the technician should place some kind of padding between the patient and the wall. Despite precautions, there have been some cases of burns being so severe that patients have needed skin grafts.
3. Hearing loss. The machines are *very, very* loud. You'll be given hearing protection, so make sure you keep it on at all times when in the room.

"It was really tight in the tunnel. So tight that there was only above six inches above my head. But it wasn't as bad as I thought it would be. Both ends were open, so it wasn't quite as claustrophobic as I thought. I was surprised that the table moved – that was a little disconcerting, but the big thing for me is that I had my husband in the room. That made me a bit calmer during the procedure (he could rescue me if I needed!)." Jill—Houston, TX.

Aortography

Although non-invasive procedures like MRI have largely replaced aortography, your physician may recommend this procedure if he suspects you have acute aortic dissection (separation of the layers within the aortic wall).

Aortic angiography is a procedure that uses a special dye and x-rays to see how blood flows through the aorta, the major artery leading out of the heart, and through your abdomen or belly.

How the Test is Performed

This test is done in a special unit of the hospital. Before the test starts, you will be given a mild sedative to help you relax.

- An area of your body, usually in your arm or groin area, is cleaned and numbed with a local numbing medicine (anesthetic).
- A radiologist or cardiologist will place a needle into the groin blood vessel. A guidewire and a long tube (catheter) will be passed through this needle.
- The catheter is carefully moved into the aorta. The doctor can see live images of the aorta on a TV-like monitor, and x-rays are used to guide the catheter to the correct position.

- Once the catheter is in place, dye is injected into it. X-ray images are taken to see how the dye moves through the aorta. The dye helps detect any blockages in blood flow.

After the x-rays or treatments are finished, the catheter is removed. Pressure is immediately applied to the puncture site for 20 - 45 minutes to stop the bleeding. After that time, the area is checked and a tight bandage is applied. The leg is usually kept straight for another 6 hours after the procedure.

How to Prepare for the Test

You will be asked not to eat or drink anything for 6-8 hours before the test.

You will be asked to wear a hospital gown and sign a consent form for the procedure. Remove jewelry from the area being studied.

Tell your health care provider:

- If you are pregnant
- If you have ever had any allergic reactions to x-ray contrast material or iodine substances
- If you are allergic to any medications
- Which medications you are taking (including any herbal preparations)

- If you have ever had any bleeding problems

How the Test will Feel

You will be awake during the test. You may feel a sting as the numbing medicine is given and some pressure as the catheter is inserted. You may feel a warm flushing when the contrast dye flows through the catheter. This is normal and usually goes away within a few seconds.

You may have some discomfort from lying on the hospital table and staying still for a long time.

Generally, you can resume normal activity the day after the procedure.

Risks

Risks of aortic angiography include:

- Allergic reaction to the contrast dye
- Blockage of the artery
- Blood clot that travels to the lungs
- Bruising at the site of catheter insertion
- Damage to the blood vessel where the needle and catheter are inserted

- Excessive bleeding or a blood clot where the catheter is inserted, which can reduce blood flow to the leg
- Heart attack or stroke
- Hematoma -- a collection of blood at the site of the needle puncture
- Infection
- Injury to the nerves at the needle puncture site
- Kidney damage from the dye

Immunohistologic evaluation of the skin (which necessitates a skin biopsy) has occasionally been used to aid in a diagnosis of MFS. However, it does come with a high number of false-positive results and so is not widely used in the US.

Many people, especially adults who are diagnosed or parents of an MFS child, find an MFS diagnosis difficult to accept and have trouble with fear, depression and even anger. If you've been recently diagnosed with MFS, consider seeing a psychotherapist or other mental health professional or reaching out to a Marfan support group if you are having difficulties in coping with your diagnosis.

Treatment

Treatment for MFS is wide and varied, depending on which body systems or organs are affected. However, there are a few general measures recommended for all MFS patients.

1. Moderate restriction of physical activity.

You should not participate in contact sports such as basketball, boxing, hockey, martial arts, soccer or wrestling. You should also avoid strenuous activities that can put stress on your aorta, like intense bicycling, gymnastics, equestrian activities, skiing or squash. You should also avoid any activity where there is a change in pressure (like scuba diving or fast elevators in high-rises). People with MFS are susceptible to a collapsed lung during these activities.

Your physical activity will depend on your overall health and any medications that you may be taking. For example, if you are taking a beta blocker to reduce stress on the aorta, this lowers your pulse at rest and makes it more difficult to achieve levels of physical fitness. Talk with your physician about what types of exercise are right for you.

If your child has MFS, make sure their school knows about their condition and limitations. Try to enroll your child in low-impact activities that they can continue as they grow into adulthood, like golf, bowling or archery.

Endocarditis prophylaxis

At one time, the American Heart Association (AHA) recommended that anyone with a mitral valve prolapse or other heart valve dysfunction take antibiotics for dental work. However, in 2007 the AHA revised those guidelines. It is now recommended that you take oral antibiotics before dental work if you have an artificial heart valve, a history of infective endocarditis, congenital heart disease or you are a heart transplant recipient. Make sure your dentist knows about your condition, and consult with your doctor about whether antibiotics prior to dental surgery are necessary for your condition.

Echocardiography

Echocardiography is recommended at least every year to check up on your heart and aorta. This may be performed every six months, especially if your physician notes changes in your heart or in young MFS patients.

Yearly checkups

You should have a physical every year so that your physician can monitor your disease. This examination should include an echocardiogram.

Specific treatments/conditions

Aortic root dilation or aortic dissection

Aortic root surgery may be considered when the diameter of your aortic root is over 5 cm or if you have aortic dissection. Several procedures may be performed, depending on what types of health issues you have and which procedures your surgical team is familiar with. For example, the Button Bentall (simultaneous replacement of the aortic valve, root and the entire ascending aorta) or David valve-sparing procedure (replacement of the aortic root and ascending aorta only) address the aortic valve and root. Button Bentall involves the insertion of a Dacron graft and is commonly used for MFS. A David Valve-Sparing procedure can be used if the dilation isn't too extreme; a Dacron graft is still implanted, but the aortic valve is not replaced – it is re-implanted inside the Dacron graft.

You can see a video of a David Procedure here: http://www.valleyheartandvascular.com/Thoracic-Aneurysm-Program/Video-of-David-Procedure.aspx

In some cases, the decision about which technique to use is sometimes made during the actual surgery. Other, less-common techniques that may be used include:

Yacoub remodeling – a procedure which creates a new aortic root out of Dracon.

Homograft technique – involves replacement of parts with tissue from a cadaver. They are generally used in older patients who have a life-expectancy of less than 15 years.

Prophylactic (preventative) surgery of the aortic root is recommended if:

1. You have a family history of aortic dissection.
2. If the aortic root grows more than 10mm per year.
3. A specific part of your heart (the aortic sinus) is dilated and it involves the ascending aorta.
4. If you have moderate aortic regurgitation or severe mitral regurgitation.

5. If you need major surgery for a non heart-related condition.
6. If you are thinking about becoming pregnant.

Several other factors may be taken into consideration for prophylactic surgery. The surgery is usually not performed until at least adolescence. It can substantially prolong your life.

Anticoagulant medications such as warfarin are taken for life after artificial heart-valve placement. Warfarin is a medication that helps to prevent blood clots.

What is a Dracon Graft?
A Dacron graft is a man-made (synthetic) material that is used to replace normal body tissues. It is usually made in a tube form to replace or repair blood vessels.

The graft causes very few reactions. It is chemically harmless and easily tolerated by the body. When used in blood vessels, the body eventually grows a new lining to the graft that mimics normal blood vessel linings.

It isn't possible to discuss major heart surgery within the scope of this book. If you are considering heart, surgery, there are many good books available on the subject. We recommend The Open Heart Companion: Preparation and Guidance for Open-Heart Surgery by Maggie Lichtenberg and Kathleen Blake.

Medications

Beta blockers

Beta blockers help to lower your blood pressure and reduce pressure on your heart. This can help slow down or even prevent aortic dilation and reduce the risk of aortic dissection. Beta-blockers are recommender for older children and adults who have MFS and an enlarged aorta. The optimal age for beta blockers hasn't been established. Some physicians will start beta blockers in infancy; others will monitor your condition until they think beta blockers are necessary. Beta-blockers slow your heart rate and put less stress on the aorta (Shores). Beta-blockers can be considered at any age if you have a dilated aorta. However, the treatment tends to be more effective if the diameter of your aorta is less than 4 cm. ACE inhibitors reduce pressure in your arteries and are sometimes recommended to be used alongside beta blockers.

Angiotensin receptor blockers (ARBs)

One particular ARB, called losartan (Cozaar®), shows promise for preventing aortic growth. At the time of writing, research is being conducted to compare the drug to beta blockers for MFS patients who cannot tolerate beta blockers.

Protrusio acetabuli

Protrusio acetabuli is a disorder of the socket in the hips. The socket is too deep and may protrude into the pelvis. Some cases may be treated with physical therapy (which involves forced stretching) although a hip graft or hip replacement surgery may be necessary.

What Is a Hip Replacement?

Hip replacement, or arthroplasty, is a surgical procedure in which the diseased parts of the hip joint are removed and replaced with new, artificial parts. These artificial parts are called the prosthesis. The goals of hip replacement surgery include increasing mobility, improving the function of the hip joint, and relieving pain. According to the Centers for Disease Control and Prevention (CDC), 332,000 total hip replacements are performed in the United States each year.

What Does Hip Replacement Surgery Involve?

The hip joint is located where the upper end of the femur, or thigh bone, meets the pelvis, or hip bone. A ball at the end of the femur, called the femoral head, fits in a socket (the acetabulum) in the pelvis to allow a wide range of motion.

During a traditional hip replacement, which lasts from 1 to 2 hours, the surgeon makes a 6- to 8-inch incision over the side of the hip through the muscles and removes the diseased bone tissue and cartilage from the hip joint, while leaving the healthy parts of the joint intact. Then the surgeon replaces the head of the femur and acetabulum with new, artificial parts. The new hip is made of materials that allow a natural gliding motion of the joint.

In recent years, some surgeons have begun performing what is called a minimally invasive, or mini-incision, hip replacement, which requires smaller incisions and a shorter recovery time than traditional hip replacement. Candidates for this type of surgery are usually age 50 or younger, of normal weight based on body mass index and healthier than candidates for traditional surgery. Joint resurfacing is also being used.

Regardless of whether you have traditional or minimally invasive surgery, the parts used to replace the joint are the same and come in two general varieties: cemented and uncemented.

Cemented parts are fastened to existing, healthy bone with a special glue or cement. Hip replacement using these parts is referred to as a "cemented" procedure. Uncemented parts rely on a process called biologic fixation, which holds them in place. This means that the parts are made with a porous surface that allows your own bone to grow into the pores and hold the new parts in place. Sometimes a doctor will use a cemented femur part and uncemented acetabular part. This combination is referred to as a hybrid replacement.

Is a Cemented or Uncemented Prosthesis Better?

The answer to this question is different for different people. Because each person's condition is unique, the doctor and you must weigh the advantages and disadvantages.

Cemented replacements are more frequently used for older, less active people and people with weak bones, such as those who have osteoporosis, while uncemented replacements are more frequently used for younger, more active people.

Studies show that cemented and uncemented prostheses have comparable rates of success. Studies also indicate that if you need an additional hip replacement, or revision, the rates of success for cemented and uncemented prostheses are comparable. However, more long-term data are available in the United States for hip replacements with cemented prostheses, because doctors have been using them here since the late 1960s, whereas uncemented prostheses were not introduced until the late 1970s.

The primary disadvantage of an uncemented prosthesis is the extended recovery period. Because it takes a long time for the natural bone to grow and attach to the prosthesis, a person with uncemented replacements must limit activities for up to 3 months to protect the hip joint. Also, it is more common for someone with an uncemented prosthesis to experience thigh pain in the months following the surgery, while the bone is growing into the prosthesis.

How to Prepare for Surgery and Recovery

People can do many things before and after they have surgery to make everyday tasks easier and help speed their recovery.

Before Surgery

- Learn what to expect. Request information written for patients from the doctor, or contact one of the organizations listed near the end of this publication.

- Arrange for someone to help you around the house for a week or two after coming home from the hospital.

- Arrange for transportation to and from the hospital.

- Set up a "recovery station" at home. Place the television remote control, radio, telephone, medicine, tissues, wastebasket, and pitcher and glass next to the spot where you will spend the most time while you recover.

- Place items you use every day at arm's level to avoid reaching up or bending down.

- Stock up on kitchen supplies and prepare food in advance, such as frozen casseroles or soups that can be reheated and served easily.

After Surgery

- Follow the doctor's instructions.

- Work with a physical therapist or other health care professional to rehabilitate your hip.

- Wear an apron for carrying things around the house. This leaves hands and arms free for balance or to use crutches.

- Use a long-handled "reacher" to turn on lights or grab things that are beyond arm's length.

Hospital personnel may provide one of these or suggest where to buy one.

What Can Be Expected Immediately After Surgery?

You will be allowed only limited movement immediately after hip replacement surgery. When you are in bed, pillows or a special device are usually used to brace the hip in the correct position. You may receive fluids through an intravenous tube to replace fluids lost during surgery. There also may be a tube located near the incision to drain fluid, and a type of tube called a catheter may be used to drain urine until you are able to use the bathroom. The doctor will prescribe medicine for pain or discomfort.

On the day after surgery or sometimes on the day of surgery, therapists will teach you exercises to improve recovery. A respiratory therapist may ask you to breathe deeply, cough, or blow into a simple device that measures lung capacity. These exercises reduce the collection of fluid in the lungs after surgery.

As early as 1 to 2 days after surgery, you may be able to sit on the edge of the bed, stand, and even walk with assistance.

While you are still in the hospital, a physical therapist may teach you exercises such as contracting and relaxing certain muscles, which can strengthen the hip. Because the new, artificial hip has a more limited range of movement than a natural, healthy hip, the physical therapist also will teach you the proper techniques for simple activities of daily living, such as bending and sitting, to prevent injury to your new hip.

How Long Are Recovery and Rehabilitation?

Usually, people do not spend more than 3 to 5 days in the hospital after hip replacement surgery. Full recovery from the surgery takes about 3 to 6 months, depending on the type of surgery, your overall health, and the success of your rehabilitation.

It is important to get instructions from your doctor before leaving the hospital and to follow them carefully once you get home. Doing so will you give you the greatest chance of a successful surgery.

What Are Possible Complications of Hip Replacement Surgery?

New technology and advances in surgical techniques have greatly reduced the risks involved with hip replacements.

The most common problem that may arise soon after hip replacement surgery is hip dislocation. Because the artificial ball and socket are smaller than the normal ones, the ball can become dislodged from the socket if the hip is placed in certain positions. The most dangerous position usually is pulling the knees up to the chest.

The most common later complication of hip replacement surgery is an inflammatory reaction to tiny particles that gradually wear off of the artificial joint surfaces and are absorbed by the surrounding tissues. The inflammation may trigger the action of special cells that eat away some of the bone, causing the implant to loosen. To treat this complication, the doctor may use anti-inflammatory medications or recommend revision surgery (replacement of an artificial joint). Medical scientists are experimenting with new materials that last longer and cause less inflammation. Less common complications of hip replacement surgery include infection, blood clots, and heterotopic bone formation (bone growth beyond the normal edges of bone).

To minimize the risk of complications, it's important to know how to prevent problems and to recognize signs of potential problems early and contact your doctor. For example, tenderness; redness and swelling of your calf; or swelling of your thigh, ankle, or foot could be warning signs of a possible blood clot. Warning signs of infection include fever, chills, tenderness and swelling, or drainage from the wound. You should call your doctor if you experience any of these symptoms.

When Is Revision Surgery Necessary?

Hip replacement is one of the most successful orthopaedic surgeries performed. However, because more people are having hip replacements at a younger age, and wearing away of the joint surface becomes a problem after 15 to 20 years, replacement of an artificial joint, which is also known as revision surgery, is becoming more common. It is more difficult than first-time hip replacement surgery, and the outcome is generally not as good, so it is important to explore all available options before having additional surgery.

Doctors consider revision surgery for two reasons: if medication and lifestyle changes do not relieve pain and disability, or if x rays of the hip show damage to the bone around the artificial hip that must be corrected before it is too late for a successful revision. This surgery is usually considered only when bone loss, wearing of the joint surfaces, or joint loosening shows up on an x ray. Other possible reasons for revision surgery include fracture, dislocation of the artificial parts, and infection.

Myopia (nearsightedness)
Myopia is treatable with refractive surgery, which can be performed in a variety of ways. A

common surgical treatment is LASIK, where a surgeon uses a laser to cut a flap through the top of your cornea. A laser is used to remove some corneal tissue, and then the flap is dropped back into place. Lasers can also be used to restore a detached retina. If your vision cannot be restored by refractive surgery, your physician may recommend that your lens is removed and replaced.

What is LASIK?

LASIK stands for Laser-Assisted *In Situ* Keratomileusis and is a procedure that permanently changes the shape of the cornea, the clear covering of the front of the eye, using an excimer laser. A mechanical microkeratome (a blade device) or a laser keratome (a laser device) is used to cut a flap in the cornea. A hinge is left at one end of this flap. The flap is folded back revealing the stroma, the middle section of the cornea. Pulses from a computer-controlled laser vaporize a portion of the stroma and the flap is replaced.

What are the risks and how can I find the right doctor for me?

Most patients are very pleased with the results of their refractive surgery. However, like any other medical procedure, there are risks involved. That's why it is important for you to understand the limitations and possible complications of refractive surgery.

Before undergoing a refractive procedure, you should carefully weigh the risks and benefits based on your own personal value system, and try to avoid being influenced by friends that have had the procedure or doctors encouraging you to do so.

- **Some patients lose vision.** Some patients lose lines of vision on the vision chart that cannot be corrected with glasses, contact lenses, or surgery as a result of treatment.
- **Some patients develop debilitating visual symptoms.** Some patients develop glare, halos, and/or double vision that can seriously affect nighttime vision. Even with good vision on the vision chart, some patients do not see as well in situations of low contrast, such as at night or in fog, after treatment as compared to before treatment.
- **You may be under treated or over treated.** Only a certain percent of patients achieve 20/20 vision without glasses or contacts. You may require additional treatment, but additional treatment may not be possible. You may still need glasses or contact lenses after surgery. This may be true even if you only required a very weak prescription before surgery. If you used reading glasses before surgery, you may still need reading glasses after surgery.

- **Some patients may develop severe dry eye syndrome.** As a result of surgery, your eye may not be able to produce enough tears to keep the eye moist and comfortable. Dry eye not only causes discomfort, but can reduce visual quality due to intermittent blurring and other visual symptoms. This condition may be permanent. Intensive drop therapy and use of plugs or other procedures may be required.
- **Results are generally not as good in patients with very large refractive errors of any type.** You should discuss your expectations with your doctor and realize that you may still require glasses or contacts after the surgery.
- **Long-term data are not available.** LASIK is a relatively new technology. The first laser was approved for LASIK eye surgery in 1998. Therefore, the long-term safety and effectiveness of LASIK surgery is not known.

Bilateral Simultaneous Treatment

You may choose to have LASIK surgery on both eyes at the same time or to have surgery on one eye at a time. Although the convenience of having surgery on both eyes on the same day is attractive, this practice is riskier than having two separate surgeries.

If you decide to have one eye done at a time, you and your doctor will decide how long to wait before having surgery on the other eye. If both eyes are treated at the same time or before one eye has a chance to fully heal, you and your doctor do not have the advantage of being able to see how the first eye responds to surgery before the second eye is treated.

Another disadvantage to having surgery on both eyes at the same time is that the vision in both eyes may be blurred after surgery until the initial healing process is over, rather than being able to rely on clear vision in at least one eye at all times.

Finding the Right Doctor

If you are considering refractive surgery, make sure you:

- **Compare.** The levels of risk and benefit vary slightly not only from procedure to procedure, but from device to device depending on the manufacturer, and from surgeon to surgeon depending on their level of experience with a particular procedure. You may want to find a doctor who is familiar with MFS.
- **Don't base your decision simply on cost** and don't settle for the first eye center, doctor, or procedure you investigate. Remember that the decisions you make about your eyes and refractive surgery will affect you for the rest of your life.
- Be wary of eye centers that advertise, "20/20 vision or your money back" or "package deals." There are **never any guarantees** in medicine.

- **Read.** It is important for you to read the patient handbook provided to your doctor by the manufacturer of the device used to perform the refractive procedure. Your doctor should provide you with this handbook and be willing to discuss his/her outcomes (successes as well as complications) compared to the results of studies outlined in the handbook.

Even the best screened patients under the care of most skilled surgeons can experience serious complications.

- **During surgery.** Malfunction of a device or other error, such as cutting a flap of cornea through and through instead of making a hinge during LASIK surgery, may lead to discontinuation of the procedure or irreversible damage to the eye.
- **After surgery.** Some complications, such as migration of the flap, inflammation or infection, may require another procedure and/or intensive treatment with drops. Even with aggressive therapy, such complications may lead to temporary loss of vision or even irreversible blindness.

Under the care of an experienced doctor, carefully screened candidates with reasonable expectations and a clear understanding of the risks and alternatives are likely to be happy with the results of their refractive procedure.

Advertising

Be cautious about "slick" advertising and/or deals that

sound "too good to be true." Remember, they usually are. There is a lot of competition resulting in a great deal of advertising and bidding for your business. Do your homework.

What should I expect before, during, and after surgery?

What to expect before, during, and after surgery will vary from doctor to doctor and patient to patient. This section is a compilation of patient information developed by manufacturers and healthcare professionals, but cannot replace the dialogue you should have with your doctor. Read this information carefully and discuss your expectations with your doctor.

Before Surgery

If you decide to go ahead with LASIK surgery, you will need an initial or baseline evaluation by your eye doctor to determine if you are a good candidate. This is what you need to know to prepare for the exam and what you should expect:

If you wear contact lenses, it is a good idea to stop wearing them **before your baseline evaluation** and switch to wearing your glasses full-time. Contact lenses change the shape of your cornea for up to several weeks after you have stopped using them depending on the type of contact lenses you wear. Not leaving your contact lenses out long enough for your cornea to assume its natural shape before surgery can have negative consequences. These consequences include inaccurate measurements and a poor surgical plan, resulting in poor vision after surgery. These measurements, which determine how much corneal tissue to remove, may need to be repeated at least a week after your initial evaluation and before surgery to make sure they have not changed, especially if you wear RGP or hard lenses. If you wear:

- **soft contact lenses**, you should stop wearing them for 2 weeks before your initial evaluation.
- **toric soft lenses or rigid gas permeable (RGP) lenses,** you should stop wearing them for at least 3 weeks before your initial evaluation.
- **hard lenses,** you should stop wearing them for at least 4 weeks before your initial evaluation.

You should tell your doctor:

- about your past and present medical and eye conditions
- about all the medications you are taking, including over-the-counter medications and any medications you may be allergic to

Your doctor should perform a **thorough eye exam** and discuss:

- whether you are a **good candidate**

- what the risks, benefits, and alternatives of the surgery are
- what you should expect before, during, and after surgery
- what your responsibilities will be before, during, and after surgery

You should have the opportunity to ask your doctor questions during this discussion. Give yourself plenty of time to think about the risk/benefit discussion, to review any informational literature provided by your doctor, and to have any additional questions answered by your doctor before deciding to go through with surgery and before signing the informed consent form.

You should not feel pressured by your doctor, family, friends, or anyone else to make a decision about having surgery. Carefully consider the pros and cons.

The **day before surgery,** you should stop using:

- creams
- lotions
- makeup
- perfumes

These products as well as debris along the eyelashes may increase the risk of infection during and after surgery. Your doctor may ask you to scrub your eyelashes for a period of time before surgery to get rid of residues and debris along the lashes.

Also **before surgery,** arrange for transportation to and from your surgery and your first follow-up visit. On the day of surgery, your doctor may give you some medicine to make you relax. Because this medicine impairs your ability to drive and because your vision may be blurry, even if you don't drive make sure someone can bring you home after surgery.

During Surgery

The surgery should take less than 30 minutes. You will lie on your back in a reclining chair in an exam room containing the laser system. The laser system includes a large machine with a microscope attached to it and a computer screen.

A numbing drop will be placed in your eye, the area around your eye will be cleaned, and an instrument called a lid speculum will be used to hold your eyelids open.

Your doctor may use a mechanical microkeratome (a blade device) to cut a flap in the cornea.

If a mechanical microkeratome is used, a ring will be placed on your eye and very high pressures will be applied to create suction to the cornea. Your vision will dim while the suction ring is on and you may feel the pressure and experience some discomfort during this part of the procedure. The microkeratome, a cutting instrument, is attached to the suction ring. Your doctor will use the blade of the microkeratome to cut a flap in your cornea. Microkeratome blades are meant to be used only once and then thrown out. The microkeratome and the suction ring are then removed.

Your doctor may use a laser keratome (a laser device), instead of a mechanical microkeratome, to cut a flap on the cornea.

If a laser keratome is used, the cornea is flattened with a clear plastic plate. Your vision will dim and you may feel the pressure and experience some discomfort during this part of the procedure. Laser energy is focused inside the cornea tissue, creating thousands of small bubbles of gas and water that expand and connect to separate the tissue underneath the cornea surface, creating a flap. The plate is then removed.

You will be able to see, but you will experience fluctuating degrees of blurred vision during the rest of the procedure. The doctor will then lift the flap and fold it back on its hinge, and dry the exposed tissue.

The laser will be positioned over your eye and you will be asked to stare at a light. This is **not** the laser used to remove tissue from the cornea. This light is to help you keep your eye fixed on one spot once the laser comes on. **NOTE: If you cannot stare at a fixed object for at least 60 seconds, you may not be a good candidate for this surgery.**

When your eye is in the correct position, your doctor will start the laser. At this point in the surgery, you may become aware of new sounds and smells. The pulse of the laser makes a ticking sound. As the laser removes corneal tissue, some people have reported a smell similar to burning hair. A computer controls the amount of laser energy delivered to your eye. Before the start of surgery, your doctor will have programmed the computer to vaporize a particular amount of tissue based on the measurements taken at your initial evaluation. After the pulses of laser energy vaporize the corneal tissue, the flap is put back into position.

A shield should be placed over your eye at the end of the procedure as protection, since no stitches are used to hold the flap in place. It is important for you to wear this shield to prevent you from rubbing your eye and putting pressure on your eye while you sleep, and to protect your eye from accidentally being hit or poked until the flap has healed.

After Surgery

Immediately after the procedure, your eye may burn, itch, or feel like there is something in it. You may experience some discomfort, or in some cases, mild pain and your doctor may suggest you take a mild pain reliever. Both your eyes may tear or water. Your vision will probably be hazy or blurry. You will instinctively want to rub your eye, but don't! Rubbing your eye could dislodge the flap, requiring further treatment. In addition, you may experience sensitivity to light, glare, starbursts or haloes around lights, or the whites of your eye may look red or bloodshot.

These symptoms should improve considerably within the first few days after surgery. You should plan on taking a few days off from work until these symptoms subside. **You should contact your doctor immediately** and not wait for your scheduled visit, if you experience severe pain, or if your vision or other symptoms get worse instead of better.

You should see your doctor within the **first 24 to 48** hours after surgery and at regular intervals after that for at least the first six months. At the first postoperative visit, your doctor will remove the eye shield, test your vision, and examine your eye. Your doctor may give you one or more types of eye drops to take at home to help prevent infection and/or inflammation. You may also be advised to use artificial tears to help lubricate the eye. Do not resume wearing a contact lens in the operated eye, even if your vision is blurry.

You should wait **one to three days** following surgery before beginning any non-contact sports, depending on the amount of activity required, how you feel, and your doctor's instructions.

To help prevent infection, you may need to wait for up to **two weeks after surgery or until your doctor advises you otherwise** before using lotions, creams, or make-up around the eye. Your doctor may advise you to continue scrubbing your eyelashes for a period of time after surgery. You should also avoid swimming and using hot tubs or whirlpools for 1-2 months.

It is important to protect your eyes from anything that might get in them and from being hit or bumped.

During the **first few months** after surgery, your vision may fluctuate.

- It may take up to three to six months for your vision to stabilize after surgery.
- Glare, haloes, difficulty driving at night, and other visual symptoms may also persist during this stabilization period. If further correction or enhancement is necessary, you should wait until your eye measurements are consistent for two consecutive visits at least 3 months apart before re-operation.
- It is important to realize that although distance vision may improve after re-operation, it is unlikely that other visual symptoms such as glare or haloes will improve.
- It is also important to note that no laser company has presented enough evidence for the FDA to make conclusions about the safety or effectiveness of enhancement surgery.

Contact your eye doctor immediately, if you develop any new, unusual or worsening symptoms at any point after surgery. Such symptoms could signal a problem that, if not treated early enough, may lead to a loss of vision.

Lens dislocation

Glasses or contact lenses can help restore vision in most cases. Fitting patients with the correct lenses is a challenge with MFS because the optician will need to decide if the glasses should work with your dislocated lens or ignore it. This can be a lengthy procedure involving trial and error. Eyedrops that dilate your pupils may also be prescribed for daily use. Surgery to implant an artificial lens is an option although most experts recommend the surgery is delayed until the eye has stopped growing in the late teens. Replacing the lens is also used for some cases of **cataracts** and other lens-related vision problems.

When is it the right time for surgery?

Whether and when to have surgery is a personal decision. It will very much depend on how much someone's vision loss is affecting their independence and everyday activities. The following factors might play an important role: How good does my eyesight have to be for me to be able to do my job? Are there certain things that I can no longer do, such as reading and sports? Do I have problems finding my way around? Is it becoming too dangerous for me to drive a car?

There is generally no reason to have surgery if a doctor has noticed that the lens is becoming cloudy but it is not yet causing any problems.

In most cases, the timing of surgery will not affect how successful the outcome is: the extent to which the cataract has progressed does not usually influence how well you can see with the newly implanted lens after surgery. But surgery is more difficult if the cataract is very advanced. Eye tests are also no longer as accurate. So it is a good idea to have regular eye tests carried out by an eye doctor (an ophthalmologist). You can then talk to him or her about the right time for surgery.

Surgery is only performed on one eye at a time. If both eyes are affected by cataracts or a dislocated lens, one eye is operated after the other.

What should I consider before having surgery?

Another factor that is important for the decision is whether or not someone has other (eye) conditions that could influence the outcome of surgery. Some people also have glaucoma, age-related macular degeneration or eye damage from diabetes. If that is the case, surgery might not clearly improve their vision.

Although most operations do not lead to complications, problems can arise. The eye doctor should thoroughly inform you about the possible advantages and disadvantages of surgery before it is carried out.

What does the surgery involve?

Surgery involves removing the lens and replacing it with an artificial lens. At the beginning of the operation, a small cut is made at the edge of the cornea (the clear covering of the eye). Next, the membrane enclosing the lens is opened at the front. The inner core and outer cortex of the lens are then broken up into small pieces using ultrasound and sucked out through a small cut (phacoemulsification). Once the old lens has been removed in this way, an artificial lens is implanted. The artificial lens lasts a lifetime. Stitches are usually not needed at the end of the operation because the cuts are so small that they normally heal quickly on their own.

The operation takes about 20 to 30 minutes. In most cases it is an outpatient procedure: you can be picked up to go home a few hours after the surgery.

People might stay in the hospital following surgery if they need more intensive care because of other conditions. Talk with your doctor about your

MFS to find out if you might have to stay in the hospital after the procedure for monitoring.

What is the most appropriate type of anesthesia?

The surgery can usually be done under local anesthetic. The anesthetic is either given as an injection next to the eye or in the form of eye drops. Both have pros and cons: studies have shown that people who have an injection generally feel less pain during and after surgery. But injections increase the risk of complications.

Pain was experienced during or after surgery by

- 360 out of 1,000 people who had eye drops and

- 130 out of 1,000 people who had an injection.

Anesthesia-related complications:

- About 80 out of 1,000 people who have an injection for cataract surgery are affected by swelling of the conjunctiva, bruising or bleeding in the eye.

- This kind of complication is much less common when eye drops are used, affecting about 1 out of 1,000 people.

The type of anesthetic used probably does not influence how good people's eyesight is after surgery.

Anesthetic eye drops do not affect the eye muscles, so it is possible to move your eyes during surgery. People are therefore asked to look in one direction and keep their eyes still throughout the procedure. Because they need to be very calm and concentrated to do this, anesthetic eye drops are not the right option for everyone, and are only considered for short operations.

How effective is surgery?

About 9 out of 10 people can see better after surgery: they see more clearly and more contrast and are able to see better in dim light too. So surgery can improve your quality of life and make everyday activities easier. Many people are able to do things that were no longer possible, or were difficult, before they had surgery – like driving a car, reading and working at a computer screen. But it can take a few weeks or months for your eyesight to improve as much as possible.

Artificial lenses usually last a lifetime and cannot wear out or become cloudy, so they generally do not have to be replaced. But sometimes a secondary cataract (also known as posterior capsule opacity) develops. This is where people's eyesight gets worse again months or years after surgery because the back of the lens capsule becomes cloudy. It is estimated that about 50 to 100 out of 1,000 people develop secondary cataracts within five years of initial cataract surgery. Secondary cataracts can be treated with a laser.

What are the possible complications?

This type of surgery does not usually cause complications. But inflammations, injuries, bleeding and wound-healing problems are possible. This can lead to vision problems that need to be treated. The most common problems are listed below.

During surgery:

- Damage to the lens capsule: in about 20 to 30 out of 1,000 cases

- Damage to the iris or eyeball: in about 1 to 5 out of 1,000 cases

After surgery:

- Swelling of the retina: in about 20 to 30 out of 1,000 cases
- Lens dislocation: in about 2 to 10 out of 1,000 cases
- Detachment of the retina: in about 2 to 10 out of 1,000 cases
- Inflammation inside of the eye (endophthalmitis): in about 1 to 2 out of 1,000 cases

Some complications are more likely if the eye is anesthetized using an injection. People who have other eye conditions have a higher risk of complications too.

Most complications do not have any long-term consequences. But they can lead to temporary problems such as impaired vision or slower wound healing. People might have to take medication for a while, or further eye surgery might be needed.

The most serious complication is an inflammation inside of the eye. This happens when germs get into the inside of the eye, causing an infection. Symptoms include pain, swelling, a red eye and severe vision problems. If these symptoms arise in the days or weeks following surgery, it is important to see an eye doctor as soon as possible. In the worst case, this kind of inflammation can lead to blindness or loss of the eye, so quick treatment with antibiotics is needed. Bleeding in the eye can cause serious complications too. But bleeding is less common than inflammations inside of the eye, affecting fewer than 1 out of 1,000 people.

How do the artificial lenses differ?

Artificial lenses are also known as intraocular lenses (IOLs). The following different types of lenses are available:

- **Monofocal lenses:** This type of lens allows clear vision at one distance. People have to decide beforehand what kind of monofocal lens they would like, depending on whether they would prefer to have clear vision when looking at things that are far away, at an intermediate distance, or nearby. They can wear glasses to help them see things at other distances. For instance, if someone chooses a lens that allows them to see things that are far away clearly, they will need glasses to read a book.

- **Multifocal lenses:** These lenses allow clear vision both when looking at things that are far away and things that are nearby. People who have multifocal lenses sometimes do not need to wear glasses at all. But their vision might still be blurred when looking at objects at certain distances, and they see somewhat less contrast than people who wear monofocal lenses. Glare is more of a problem with multifocal lenses too, for example when driving at night.

- **Toric lenses:** This type of lens is especially suitable for people who have astigmatism.

Multifocal lenses and toric lenses are more expensive than monofocal lenses. If patients would like to have multifocal or toric lenses, they may have to pay the difference themselves. Because using these types of lenses can be expensive, it is worth carefully weighing the pros and cons of the different types of lenses before making a decision. It might be helpful to get a second opinion from a different eye doctor.

One thing that is more important than the type of lens is the strength (the refractive power) of the lens. The lens must have the right strength for your eye. The eye doctor will do the necessary tests before the operation.

What happens after surgery?

An eye patch should be worn for one day following surgery. The eye might itch, hurt a little, and it might feel like you have something in your eye. These things usually go away again after a few days. Because the eye was recently operated on, it is important not to push on it or rub it, but it is okay to touch it gently. You can return to most everyday activities as usual after a few days, apart from driving a car. It is best to talk to your eye doctor about whether or not to avoid certain activities at first. The doctor will also let you know when your eyesight is good enough for you to start driving again. This is usually possible after a few weeks.

Eye drops are prescribed to be used for some time following surgery, and further follow-up care appointments with your eye doctor are made. Glasses can only be adjusted several weeks after surgery.

If you are thinking about eye surgery...

Make sure your eye surgeon has experience with MFS patients, as you stand a risk of more complications from lens replacement surgery. There are two types of lens replacement (posterior or anterior) and each has their pros and cons. For example, it is easier to surgically implant a lens in the anterior chamber but the lenses may be too small for

MFS patient. Posterior chamber is more difficult but may allow for a better fit. Additionally, there is a higher risk of retinal detachment during posterior chamber surgery. Which technique your eye doctor chooses is usually a matter of their personal choice. Ask your doctor about their reasons for using which type of surgery.

Flat feet (pes planus)

If you have flat feet, you may be able to treat the condition by wearing shoes that have adequate arch support. Sometimes, your doctor may recommend custom orthotics (shoe inserts which are molded to the shape of your feet). Arch supports or custom orthotics don't cure flat feet, but they may help with symptoms which can include knee pain.

Scoliosis

A brace, usually worn for 23 hours a day, is removed only for bathing, showering or swimming. The brace can prevent mild from moderate scoliosis from getting worse, but it cannot treat existing scoliosis or return the spine to "normal." It's worn until growth has stopped, about 14 or 15 for girls and 16 or 17 for boys. How successful the brace is depends on how sever the scoliosis is. For curves over 25 degrees, surgery is usually needed at some point. In fact, a brace is ineffective for treating severe scoliosis.

You may require surgery for your scoliosis if you are experiencing pain, neurological symptoms or if the curve is extreme (extreme curves over 40 degrees can cause restrictive lung disease). Scoliosis surgery usually isn't performed in children younger than 4 because of the high risk of heart complications. The surgery is performed by straightening the spine and placing metal rods underneath the back muscles. Complications, like the spine not fusing or nerve damage, are rare.

Pectus excavatum

Pectus excavatum can cause problems with the function of your heart and lungs if it is severe. Surgery, if deemed necessary, is usually delayed until mid-adolescence until the shape stabilizes. Surgery consists of raising the breastbone and ribs and straightening them. The ribs are held in place with a metal bar, which is removed after about 4 to 6 months in an outpatient procedure. Pectus carinatum (a sticking out chest) can be repaired for cosmetic reasons

Pectus excavatum repair

Pectus excavatum repair is surgery to correct pectus excavatum.

Description

There are two types of surgery to repair this condition -- open surgery and closed (minimally invasive) surgery. Both of these are done under general anesthesia.

Open surgery is more traditional. In this method, the surgeon makes a cut across the front part of the chest.

- The surgeon removes the deformed cartilage and leaves the rib lining in place. This will allow the cartilage to grow back correctly.
- The surgeon makes a cut in the breastbone and moves it aside. The surgeon may use a rib or a metal strut (support piece) to hold the breastbone in this normal position until it heals. Healing will take 3 to 6 months.
- The surgeon may place a chest tube to drain fluids that build up in the area.
- Metal struts will be removed in 6 months through a small cut in the skin under the arm. This procedure is usually done on an outpatient basis.

The second type of surgery is a closed, less invasive method (Nuss repair). It is used mostly for children. No cartilage or bone is removed.

- The surgeon makes two small cuts, one on each side of the chest. A curved steel bar that has been shaped to fit the child is inserted through the cuts and placed under the sternum (breastbone).
- This bar is guided into position using a small video camera called a thoracoscope. This camera is placed inside the chest and removed after surgery.
- Then the surgeon uses a special instrument to rotate the bar and lift the sternum or breastbone. No bone or cartilage is removed. The bar is left in place for at least 2 years.

The surgery may take 1 to 4 hours.

Why the Procedure is Performed

The most common reason for pectus excavatum repair is to improve the appearance of children who feel very self-conscious about the sunken look of their chest wall. Sometimes the deformity is so severe that it affects breathing, especially in adults later in life.

Some people may have difficulty exercising or pain that comes and goes.

Surgery is usually not done before age 6. Best results are seen when the surgery is done before adulthood.

Surgery is usually done on children who are 12 to 16 years old. It can also be done on adults in their early 20s.

Risks

The risks for any anesthesia are:

- Reactions to medicines
- Breathing problems

The risks for any surgery are:

- Bleeding
- Infection
- Scarring

Risks for this surgery are:

- Injury to the heart
- Lung collapse
- Pain
- Return of the deformity

Before the Procedure

All patients need to have a complete medical exam and a variety of tests before the surgery. The surgeon will perform the following:

- A complete medical history and physical exam

- Chest measurements and photos of the chest
- An electrocardiogram (ECG) or echocardiogram (echo) that shows how the heart is functioning
- Pulmonary function tests (PFTs) to check for any breathing problems
- Computed tomography (CT scan) or magnetic resonance imaging (MRI) of the chest to look at the internal structures below the chest

Always tell your doctor or nurse:

- What drugs you are taking. Include drugs, herbs, vitamins, or any other supplements you bought without a prescription.
- About any allergies you may have to medicine, latex, tape, or skin cleaner

During the days before the surgery:

- About 10 days before surgery, you may be asked to stop taking aspirin, ibuprofen (Advil, Motrin), naproxen (Aleve, Naprosyn), warfarin (Coumadin), and any other drugs that make it hard for blood to clot.
- Ask your doctor which drugs you should still take on the day of surgery.

On the day of the surgery:

- You will usually be asked not to drink or eat anything after midnight the night before surgery.
- Take any drugs your doctor told you to give with a small sip of water.
- Your doctor or nurse will tell you when to arrive at the hospital.
- The doctor will make sure you have no signs of illness before surgery. If you are ill, the surgery may be delayed.

After the Procedure

It is common for you to stay in the hospital for 1 week. How long you stay will probably depend on the level of discomfort after surgery.

Pain is common after the surgery. For the first few days, you may receive strong pain medicine in the vein (through an IV) or through a catheter placed in the spine (an epidural). After that, pain is usually managed with medicines taken by mouth.

You may have tubes in the chest around the surgical cuts. These tubes drain extra fluid that builds up and help the lungs expand. The tubes will remain in place until they stop draining, usually after a few days.

The day after surgery, you will be encouraged to sit up, take deep breaths, and get out of bed and walk. These activities will help healing.

At first, you will not be able to bend, twist, or roll from side to side. Activities will slowly be increased.

When you can walk without help, he or she is probably ready to go home. Before leaving the hospital, you will receive a prescription for pain medicine.

Outlook (Prognosis)

Improvements in appearance are usually good. Improvements in breathing or ability to exercise varies from patient to patient.

Pneumothorax (collapsed lung)

Placement of a chest tube is usually the first line of treatment and can restore function to your lung. The tube remains in place until your lung heals. However, there is a high risk of recurrence so surgery is usually recommended. The surgery is called thoracoscopy, bleb resection, and talc pleurodesis. With thoracoscopy, a small camera called an endoscope is put into the chest and the bleb (a blister-like pocket of air) is introduced into the chest and the bleb is removed with a surgical tool. A pleurodesis is a procedure that "glues" the lung onto the chest wall.

What does lung surgery involve?

You will receive general anesthesia before surgery. You will be asleep and unable to feel pain. Two common ways to do surgery on your lungs are thoracotomy and video-assisted thoracoscopic surgery (VATS).

Lung surgery using a thoracotomy is called open surgery. In this surgery:

- You will lie on your side on an operating table. Your arm will be placed above your head.
- Your surgeon will make a surgical cut between two ribs. The cut will go from the front of your chest wall to your back, passing just underneath the armpit. These ribs will be separated.
- Your lung on this side will be deflated so that air will not move in and out of it during surgery. This makes it easier for the surgeon to operate on the lung.
- After surgery, one or more drainage tubes will be placed into your chest area to drain out fluids that build up. These tubes are called chest tubes.

- After the surgery on your lungs, your surgeon will close the ribs, muscles, and skin with sutures.
- Open lung surgery may take from 2 to 6 hours.

Video-assisted thoracoscopic surgery:

- Your surgeon will make several small surgical cuts over your chest wall. A videoscope (a tube with a tiny camera on the end) and other small tools will be passed through these cuts.
- One or more tubes will be placed into your chest to drain fluids that build up.
- This procedure leads to much less pain and a faster recovery than open lung surgery.

However, sometimes video surgery may not be possible, and the surgeon may have to switch to an open surgery.

Risks

Risks for any anesthesia include:

- Allergic reactions to medicines
- Breathing problems

Risks for any surgery include:

- Bleeding
- Blood clots in the legs that may travel to the lungs
- Heart attack or stroke during surgery
- Infection, including in the surgical cut, lungs, bladder, or kidney

Risks of this surgery include:

- Failure of the lung to expand
- Injury to the lungs or blood vessels
- Need for a chest tube after surgery
- Pain
- Prolonged air leak
- Repeated fluid buildup in the chest cavity

Before the Procedure

Smoking isn't recommended if you have MFS. However, if you do smoke, you should stop smoking several weeks before your surgery. Ask your doctor or nurse for help.

Always tell your doctor or nurse:

- What drugs, vitamins, herbs, and other supplements you are taking, even ones you bought without a prescription

- If you have been drinking a lot of alcohol, more than 1 or 2 drinks a day

During the week before your surgery:

- You may be asked to stop taking drugs that make it hard for your blood to clot. Some of these are aspirin, ibuprofen (Advil, Motrin), vitamin E, warfarin (Coumadin), clopidogrel (Plavix), or ticlopidine (Ticlid).
- Ask your doctor which drugs you should still take on the day of your surgery.
- Prepare your home for your return from the hospital.

On the day of your surgery:

- Do not eat or drink anything after midnight the night before your surgery.
- Take the medications your doctor prescribed with small sips of water.
- Your doctor or nurse will tell you when to arrive at the hospital.

After the Procedure

Most people stay in the hospital for 5 to 7 days for open thoracotomy and 1 to 3 days after video-assisted thoracoscopic surgery. You may spend time in the intensive care unit (ICU) after either surgery.

During your hospital stay, you will:

- Be asked to sit on the side of the bed and walk as soon as possible after surgery
- Have tube(s) coming out of the side of your chest to drain fluids
- Wear special stockings on your feet and legs to prevent blood clots
- Receive shots to prevent blood clots
- Receive pain medicine through an IV (a tube that goes into your veins) or by mouth with pills. You may receive your pain medicine through a special machine that gives you a dose of pain medicine when you push a button. This allows you to control how much pain medicine you get.
- Be asked to do a lot of deep breathing to help prevent pneumonia and infection. Deep breathing exercises also help inflate the lung that was operated on. Your chest tube(s) will remain in place until your lung has fully inflated.

Pregnancy and MFS

If you or your partner have MFS, you have a 50% chance of passing the gene to your child. If both parents are affected, you have a 75% chance your child will have MFS. Also, with both parents affected, there is a chance your child could be affected with homozygous Marfan syndrome, which a potentially more serious condition; in homozygous Marfan syndrome, *both* copies of the FBN1 gene are affected. One case of homozygous MFS reported in the literature ended in an early death for the child.

Something else to consider if you have MFS and are thinking of getting pregnant: your child may have a more serious or less serious form of the disease than you, so it's essential to prepare yourself for all possibilities. Talk with a genetic counselor before you get pregnant so that you can evaluate the risk of passing MFS to your potential children.

If you are thinking of getting pregnant but do not want your child to have MFS, In Vitro Fertilization (IVF) may be an option. With IVF, the embryos are tested for Marfan syndrome before implantation. Only those embryos lacking the gene are selected for implantation. IVF can be prohibitively expensive and requires that you have already been genetically tested and that the particular mutation has been identified. IVF implantation is far from an exact science and it could take many rounds of implantation to secure a successful pregnancy. At the time of writing, the average couple going through IVF spends about $20,000. Each additional cycle costs around $7,000.

A second option is to get pregnant and have your fetus tested for MFS using prenatal testing like chorionic villus sampling or amniocentesis. Prenatal testing is possible if you have MFS and if the specific gene affected is known. Prenatal testing is carried out around 10-12 weeks gestation using chorionic villus sampling (CVS) or about 16-18 weeks gestation using amniocentesis. CVS involves taking a small sample of cells from the placenta, while amniocentesis involves taking a sample of amniotic fluid (the fluid that surrounds the baby in the womb). Although prenatal testing can tell you if your baby has MFS or not, it cannot tell you how serious the condition is. Additionally, the testing procedure is not perfect, so a negative result does not always mean your baby will not be born without MFS.

If your fetus tests positive for MFS, you then have to face the choice of keeping the child or having an abortion. This can be a difficult decision, and one that you should discuss with your physician or a mental health professional before you get pregnant.

If you have MFS and you are thinking of becoming pregnant, it can also mean a high risk pregnancy, especially if your aortic root diameter is more than 4cm. Your physician may recommend aortic root replacement if you intend to get pregnant and your aortic root is over 4cm.

If you are pregnant, you'll be closely monitored during your pregnancy, and you'll likely have several echocardiograms during your pregnancy and for three months postpartum. Even if you don't have aortic root dilation of more than 4cm, being pregnant can place additional stress on your heart and blood vessels, running the possibility that it could make any existing dilation worse. If you do have aortic disease or significant heart valve problems you should discuss risks and complications of a pregnancy before you get pregnant.

If you have had heart surgery and are taking warfarin, discuss the risks with your doctor. Warfarin poses significant risks to a fetus, especially during the first trimester (weeks 7-11) because warfarin is known to cause birth defects. It should also not be taken for about a month before delivery due to an increased risk of hemorrhage. It may be possible to place you on an alternate medication (heparin) during this time that does not cross the placenta.

Many other drugs taken for MFS, such as losartan and angiotensin converting enzyme inhibitors like enalapri, can result in birth defects. In addition, you may not be able to take certain medications during breastfeeding. Discuss all of your medications with your physician before making the decision to get pregnant.

Related disorders

Loeys-Dietz Syndrome

Loeys-Dietz Syndrome is another connective-tissue disorder which has many features in common with Marfan syndrome. In fact, it has so many features in common with MFS that it was once called (prior to about 2006) Marfan Syndrome Type II. It is more lethal than MFS and carries a high risk of aortic aneurysms and complications during pregnancy. The genes affected are TGFBR1, TGFBR2 or SMAD3. There are three types of the syndrome.

Loeys-Dietz Syndrome Type I is characterized by an enlarged aorta, which may lead to aortic dissection or aortic aneurysm. Like MFS, Loeys-Dietz Syndrome Type I patients may also have aneurysms or dissections in other parts of the body. Arteries may

have abnormal twists and turns, a condition called arterial tortuosity. Other conditions associated with Type I include:
- Widely spaced eyes
- A split in the soft flap of tissue at the back of the mouth
- Cleft palate (an opening in the roof of the mouth)
- A tendency to bruise easily and develop abnormal scars
- Premature fusion of the skull bones
- Scoliosus
- Pectus excavatum or pectus carinatum
- Club feet
- Elongated limbs with joint deformities

Loeys-Dietz Syndrome Type II has many of the features of Type I, such as arterial tortuosity, an enlarged aorta, a tendency to bruise easily and abnormal scarring. Skeletal problems tend not to be so severe. Skin problems characterize this type: skin may be velvety and translucent, so that the underlying veins are visible.

Loeys-Dietz Syndrome Type III is characterized by aortic and arterial aneurysms plus osteoarthritis (pain in the joints). This type is sometimes called aneurysms-osteoarthritis syndrome.

Ehlers-Danlos Syndrome

Ehlers-Danlos Syndrome also affects the connective tissues, but unlike MFS, the joint and skin problems are due to issues with collagen, proteins that stabilize the connective tissue and give it elasticity. Prior to 1997, there were 10 recognized types of EDS, but this has now been simplified to six major types: the arthrochalasia type, the classic type, the dermatosparaxis type, the hypermobility type, the kyphoscoliosis type, and the vascular type. Each type has its own features, although all types have some effect on the joints. For example, the vascular type of Ehlers-Danlos syndrome carries an increased risk of organ rupture, including tearing of the intestine and rupture of the uterus (womb) during pregnancy. The genes associated with the condition are *ADAMTS2*, *COL1A1*, *COL1A2*, *COL3A1*, *COL5A1*, *COL5A2*, *PLOD1*, and *TNXB*.

Ectopia Lentis Syndrome

People who inherit the skeletal features of MFS (like a tall thin body type and long arms and fingers) but do not have any other features of MFS such as aortic dilation may be diagnosed with ectopic lentis syndrome (sometimes called familial ectopia lentis) if they have lens dislocation of the eye. The only way a diagnosis can be made between the two syndromes is by frequent monitoring (i.e. echocardiograms) to rule out Marfan syndrome.

Beals Syndrome (Congenital contractural arachnodactyly)

Like MFS, Beals syndrome is an inherited connective tissue disorder with an autosomal dominant pattern of inheritance. For many years, it was thought that Beals syndrome and Marfan syndrome were the same disorder until the discovery that the two disorders were caused by mutations in different genes; Marfan syndrome is caused by a mutation in the FBN1 gene and Beals is caused by mutations in the FBN2 gene. It shares some common characteristics with MFS, including arachnodactyl, kyphoscoliosis, a highly arched palate, myopia and mitral valve prolapse. In very rare cases, people with Beals syndrome may also have aortic dilation. However, there are many features not seen in MFS, including permanently fixed fingers (camptodactyl), "crumpled" ears and permanently fixed joints in a flexed position. Beals syndrome is extremely rare, but how many people are affected is not known.

Familial Thoracic Aortic Aneurysm and Dissection (Familial TAAD)

Familial TAAD is a disorder usually involving the upper part of the aorta (the thoracic aorta). In some cases, the abdominal aorta may be affected or individuals may have brain aneurysms. People with TAAD can have aortic dilation, aneurysms and aortic dissection. However, unlike MFS, no other symptoms are usually involved with familial TAAD. Rarely, people with familial TAAD might have scoliosis, a purplish skin coloration or a pouching in the lower abdomen (inguinal hernia).

Fragile X Syndrome

Fragile X syndrome is a genetic disorder that causes many developmental problems such as cognitive impairment and learning disabilities. Individuals who have fragile X may also have heart problems like aortic root dilation or mitral valve prolapse (Sreeram) and joint laxity (Dietz). However, MFS does not cause the types of developmental problems seen in Fragile X.

Gigantism and Acromegaly

Gigantism and acromegaly both cause excessive growth. They are both caused by the production of too much growth hormone. Gigantism causes a high linear growth, resulting in a tall stature while acromegaly causes the bones to increase in size. Acromegaly usually affects middle-aged people while gigantism is seen in childhood and can co-exist with Marfan syndrome. Untreated gigantism and acromegaly can lead to heart problems, including heart failure due to an enlarged heart.

Hyperpituitarism

Hyperpituitarism is an overactive pituitary gland. The pituitary gland plays a role in a wide variety of biological functions, including metabolism, growth, sexual function and blood pressure. Three hormones are oversecreted, including <u>adrenocorticotropic hormone</u> (ACTH). Excess ACTH can result in gigantism.

Hyperthyroidism

Hyperthyroidism is where your thyroid gland produces too much of a hormone called thyroxine. Symptoms include weight loss, sweating, a rapid or irregular heartbeat and nervousness and irritability. It is not a genetic disorder but can be a differential diagnosis for MFS. A differential diagnosis is a diagnostic method to identify the presence of a disease or disorder where several others are possible.

Klinefelter Syndrome

Klinefelter syndrome is a genetic disorder that only affects males. It affects the X chromosome, but it is not inherited. Small testes that don't produce as much testosterone as usual is characteristic of the condition. Like MFS, people with this syndrome tend to be taller than their peers. However, Klinefelter causes a wide range of symptoms that are not associated with MFS, including reproductive issues, breast enlargement and delayed or incomplete puberty.

Bicuspid Aortic Valve

A Bicuspid aortic valve is an aortic valve that has two leaflets instead of the normal three. Like MFS, it can cause an enlarged aorta. However, no other MFS-like symptoms and signs are associated with this disorder. It is the most common congenital heart disease and it often runs in families.

MASS Phenotype

Like MFS, MASS phenotype is a disorder of connective tissues in the FBN1 gene. MASS stands for Mitral valve, Aorta, Skin and Skeletal. People with MASS phenotype may have mitral valve prolapsed, a large aortic root diameter, stretch marks on the skin and Marfan-like skeletal features including scoliosis, pectus excavatum or pectus carinatum. However, people with MASS syndrome do not have lens dislocation in the eye or a progression of aortic root dilation to aneurysms or the potential for aortic root dissection.

Schprintzen-Goldberg Syndrome

People with Schprintzen-Goldberg Syndrome have many Marfan-like features, including arachnodactyly, very long limbs, pectus excavatum, pectus carinatum and scoliosis. However, people Schprintzen-Goldberg Syndrome often have delayed development and mild to moderate intellectual disability. They may also have distinctive facial features including widely spaced eyes, protruding eyes, a small lower jaw and ears that are rotated back and low set. This syndrome is caused by mutations in the SKI gene.

Stickler Syndrome

Stickler syndrome is a group of hereditary conditions characterized by a distinctive, flattened facial appearance, eye abnormalities, hearing loss, and joint problems. Like MFS, Stickler syndrome can cause retinal detachment, loose joints, scoliosis and kyphosis. Other features of Stickler syndrome that are not seen in MFS include hearing loss.

Clinical Trials

Researchers are studying a variety of drugs including ACE inhibitors, angiotensin receptor blockers (ARBs) such as losartan and calcium channel blockers (such as verapamil), as alternatives to therapy with beta-blockers.
Information on government-funded clinical trials – as well as some privately funded trials -- is posted at www.clinicaltrials.gov.

Clinical trials are also being conducted at the NIH Clinical Center in Bethesda, MD.

Tollfree: (800) 411-1222
TTY: (866) 411-1010
Email: prpl@cc.nih.gov

Clinical trials sponsored by private sources are generally posted at:
www.centerwatch.com

Contact for additional information about Marfan syndrome:

Hal Dietz, MD
Victor A. McKusick Professor of Medicine and Genetics
Investigator, Howard Hughes Medical Institute
Institute of Genetic Medicine
Departments of Pediatrics, Medicine, and Molecular Biology & Genetics
Johns Hopkins University School of Medicine
733 N. Broadway, BRB 539
Baltimore, MD 21205
(410) 614-0701
(410) 614-2256 (fax)
hdietz@jhmi.edu

Marfan Syndrome Related Organizations

- American Heart Association
  - 8200 Brookriver Drive
  - Suite N-100
  - Dallas, TX 75247
  - Phone #: 214-784-7212
  - 800 #: 800-242-8721
  - e-mail: Review.personal.info@heart.org
  - Home page: http://www.americanheart.org
- Canadian Marfan Association
  - Centre Plaza Postal Outlet
  - 128 Queen Street South
  - P.O. Box 42257
  - Mississauga
  - Ontario, L5M 4Z0 Canada

- Phone #: (90-5)--826-3223
- 800 #: 866--72-2-1722
- e-mail: info@marfan.ca
- Home page: http://www.marfan.ca
- Cleft Lip and Palate Foundation of Smiles
  - 2044 Michael Ave SW
  - Wyoming, MI 49509
  - Phone #: N/A
  - 800 #: N/A
  - e-mail: Rachelmancuso09@comcast.net
  - Home page: http://www.cleftsmile.org
- Coalition for Heritable Disorders of Connective Tissue (CHDCT)
  - 4301 Connecticut Avenue, NW Suite 404
  - Washington, DC 20008
  - Phone #: 202-362-9599
  - 800 #: 800-778-7171
  - e-mail: chdct@pxe.org
  - Home page: http://www.chdct.org
- Genetic and Rare Diseases (GARD) Information Center
  - PO Box 8126
  - Gaithersburg, MD 20898-8126
  - Phone #: 301-251-4925
  - 800 #: 888-205-2311
  - e-mail: N/A
  - Home page: http://rarediseases.info.nih.gov/GARD/AboutGARD.aspx
- Madisons Foundation

- PO Box 241956
- Los Angeles, CA 90024
- Phone #: 310-264-0826
- 800 #: N/A
- e-mail: getinfo@madisonsfoundation.org
- Home page: http://www.madisonsfoundation.org
- National Marfan Foundation
  - 22 Manhasset Avenue
  - Port Washington, NY 11050
  - Phone #: 516-883-8712
  - 800 #: 800-862-7326
  - e-mail: staff@marfan.org
  - Home page: http://www.marfan.org
- National Scoliosis Foundation
  - 5 Cabot Place
  - Stoughton, MA 02072
  - Phone #: 781-341-8333
  - 800 #: 800-673-6922
  - e-mail: nsf@scoliosis.org
  - Home page: http://www.scoliosis.org
- NIH/National Institute of Arthritis and Musculoskeletal and Skin Diseases
  - Information Clearinghouse
  - One AMS Circle
  - Bethesda, MD 20892-3675 USA
  - Phone #: 301-495-4484
  - 800 #: 877-226-4267
  - e-mail: NIAMSinfo@mail.nih.gov

- Home page: http://www.niams.nih.gov/

GLOSSARY

Abdominal aortic aneurysms (AAAs): an aneurysm that occurs in the abdominal part of the aorta.
Acetabulum: part of the hip socket that receives the femoral head.
Acquired mutation: when a mistake is made when the DNA copies itself during development.
Acromegaly: a condition that causes the bones to increase in size.
Acromicric dysplasia: a disorder associated with a very short stature, short limbs, stiff joints, and distinctive facial features.

Acute aortic valvular insufficiency: a condition that results in a sudden increase of blood to the left ventricle of the heart.
Adventitia: part of the artery that is a protective outside layer.
Amblyopia: lazy eye.
Amino acid: building blocks of proteins.
Amniocentesis: a prenatal test that involves taking a sample of amniotic fluid (the fluid that surrounds the baby in the womb).
Aneurysm: a balloon-like bulge in an artery.
Angiotensin receptor blockers (ARBs): a medication that may prevent aortic growth.
Aortic dilation: where the aorta becomes enlarged.
Aortic dissection: a tear in the aorta where blood penetrates the intima and enters the media layer. The high pressure rips the tissue of the media apart.
Aortic dissection: tearing of the walls of the aorta.
Aortic root replacement: surgery to replace the aorta.
Aortography: a procedure that uses a special dye and x-rays to see how blood flows through the aorta.
Arachnodactly: abnormally slender fingers.
Arrhythmias: irregular heartbeats.
Arteries: oxygen-rich blood vessels, carrying oxygen to different parts of your body.
Ascending aorta: the part of the aorta closest to the heart.
Astigmatism: blurred vision.
Autosomal dominant: means that you only have to get the gene from one parent to be affected.

Bacterial endocarditis: a condition where bacteria in the bloodstream infect the heart valves.
Base pair: formed of two chemical bases which are bonded to each other forming a "rung of the DNA ladder."
Beta blockers: medication that helps to lower your blood pressure and reduce pressure on your heart.
Bicuspid Aortic Valve: an aortic valve that has two leaflets instead of the normal three.
Brain aneurysm is an abnormal bulge or "ballooning" in the wall of an artery in the brain.
Bunions: excessive bone growth near the base of the big toes.
Button Bentall: a procedure for simultaneous replacement of the aortic valve, root and the entire ascending aorta.
Cardiologist: a heart doctor.
Cardiovascular: heart and blood vessels.
Cataract: a clouding of the lens of the eye.
Chorionic villus sampling (CVS): a prenatal test that involves taking a small sample of cells from the placenta.
Collagen: proteins that stabilize the connective tissue and give it elasticity.
Congenital contractures: a condition where the muscles are shortened or contracted.
Connective tissue: holds all the organs, tissues and cells in your body together like glue.
Cornea: the outer part of the eye.

Cytogenetic location: refers to where a particular band of a lab-stained chromosome lies.
Dacron graft: a man-made (synthetic) material that is used to replace normal body tissues.
David valve-sparing procedure: replacement of the aortic root and ascending aorta.
De novo mutation: a mutation that occurs in either an egg or a sperm.
Descending aorta: the part of the aorta that goes down into the chest cavity and below the waist.
Diagnosis of exclusion: where physician will consider many other disorders and syndromes.
Dura: the membrane that surrounds the brain and spinal cord.
Dural ecstasia: a widening or ballooning of the sac around the spinal cord.
Ectopia lens: a dislocated lens.
Ehlers-Danlos Syndrome: a condition that also affects the connective tissues, due to issues with collagen.
Emphysema: a condition where the walls of the lungs are damaged and they cannot push all of the air out of the lungs.
Endocarditis prophylaxis: preventative treatment with antibiotics for people with certain heart problems.
Endothelial cells: the thin layer of cells that lines the interior surface of blood vessels and lymphatic vessels.
Enophthalmos: sunken in eyeballs.

Esophagus: the tube that leads from your mouth to your stomach.
Extracellular matrix: an elaborate network of proteins and molecules that fills the spaces in between the cells.
Familial thoracic aortic aneurysm and dissection (FTAAD): A hereditary disorder that causes thoracic aortic aneurysm and dissection.
FBN1 haplotype: a group of alleles that are located close to each other on the FBN1 gene and tend to be inherited together.
FBN1: the gene tells the body how to make the fibrillin-1 protein.
Fibrillin-1 protein: responsible for strengthening the body's connective tissue.
First degree relatives: close family members: parents, siblings and your children.
Fragile X Syndrome: a genetic disorder that causes many developmental problems such as cognitive impairment and learning disabilities.
Genetic map: describes where genes are found on a chromosome.
Genetic testing: a procedure that identifies exactly which mutation is present in a gene. It can also track the gene through any particular family.
Germline mutations: see hereditary mutations.
Ghent criteria: The most recent set of criteria for diagnosing MFS.
Gigantism: a disorder that causes a high linear growth, resulting in a tall stature.

Hemorrhage: a condition where the patient bleeds too much.
Hereditary mutations: Gene mutations that are passed from one of your parents.
Homograft technique – involves replacement of parts with tissue from a cadaver.
Hyperpituitarism: an overactive pituitary gland. The pituitary gland.
Hyperthyroidism: a condition where your thyroid gland produces too much of a hormone called thyroxine.
In-frame deletions: where a part of the gene is deleted
Insertion mutations: insert new DNA into the wrong place in the gene.
Intima: part of the artery in direct contact with the blood inside the vessel.
Klinefelter Syndrome: a genetic disorder that only affects males. Causes reproductive issues, breast enlargement and delayed or incomplete puberty.
Kyphosis: a hunched back of more than 45 degrees.
LASIK: surgery, where a surgeon uses a laser to cut a flap through the top of your cornea.
Leaflet: the flap in the mitral valve.
Lens: a transparent structure located behind the iris that helps to focus on objects.
Loeys-Dietz Syndrome: a connective-tissue disorder which has many features in common with Marfan syndrome.

Marfan syndrome Type II: old name for Loeys-Dietz syndrome.
Marfan Syndrome: a genetic disorder that affects the body's connective tissue.
Marfanoid habitus: a constellation of symptoms resembling those of Marfan syndrome, including long limbs, arachnodactyly, and hyperlaxity.
Marfanoid: *see* Marfanoid habitus.
MASS syndrome: which causes abnormalities in several parts of the body, including the mitral valve, the aorta, the skeleton, and the skin.
Media: part of the artery that contains connective and muscle tissue.
Medical geneticist: a physician whose specialty is genetic disorders.
Microfibrils: form elastic fibers that allow the blood vessels, skin, and ligaments to stretch.
Missense mutations. A missense mutation is when a single base pair changes.
Mitral insufficiency: a disorder where the mitral valve does not close properly.
Mitral valve prolapse (MVP): a "floppy" mitral valve that doesn't close properly.
Mitral valve regurgitation: see Mitral insufficiency.
MRI: a safe, painless technique to produce detailed 3-D images of your body.
Myopia: severe nearsightedness.
Ocular: the eyes.
Overbites: a condition where the lower jaw recedes.
Palate: the roof of the mouth.

Pectus carinatum: a chest that sticks out.
Pectus excavatum: a chest that sinks in.
Pericardial tamponade: where fluid collects in the sac surrounding the heart.
Pericardiocentesis: surgery to repair pericardial tamponade.
Pes planus: flat feet.
Prophylactic: preventative.
Protrusio acetabulae: a defect of the acetabulum.
Restrictive Lung Disease: a disease that restricts the expansion of the lungs and makes it difficult to take breaths.
Retina: the light-sensitive membrane in the back of your eye.
Schprintzen-Goldberg Syndrome: people with Schprintzen-Goldberg Syndrome have many Marfan-like features, including arachnodactyly, very long limbs, pectus excavatum, pectus carinatum and scoliosis.
Scoliosis: a spine that curves to the left or right, usually in a spiral or S-shape.
Sleep apnea: a condition that interrupts your sleep.
Weill-Marchesani syndrome: a connective tissue disorder. An eye disorder called microspherophakia is associated with this syndrome. Microspherophakia refers to a small, sphere-shaped lens.
Slit lamp machine: an eye exam machine that shines a bright light into the eye.

Spontaneous Pneumothorax: an abnormal collection of gas or air in the space between the lung and the chest wall that collapses the lung.
Stickler Syndrome: a group of hereditary conditions characterized by a distinctive, flattened facial appearance, eye abnormalities, hearing loss, and joint problems.
Stiff skin syndrome: characterized by very hard, thick skin covering most of the body.
Strabismus: where two eyes do not focus on an object at the same time.
TGFβR1: Transforming Growth Factor-Beta Receptor, Type I.
TGFβR2: Transforming Growth Factor-Beta Receptor, Type II.
The "Thumb sign": can also be used to aid a diagnosis for MFS.
Thoracic aortic aneurysm (TAA): An aneurysm that occurs in the chest part of the aorta.
Transesophageal echocardiography (TEE): a diagnostic procedure where a flexible tube with a probe at the tip is guides down your esophagus.
Transforming growth factor beta (TGF-β): helps to control growth and development.
Warfarin: an anticoagulant medication.
Yacoub remodeling: a procedure which creates a new aortic root out of Dracon.
Z-scores: used in statistics to measure how far from the mean (the average) a certain score is. In pediatric cardiology, z-scores can tell a physician how far a

patient's aorta size is from what would be expected in the "average" person of that age, height and weight.

REFERENCES

AHA guidelines J Am Dent Assoc, Vol 138, No 6, 739-760.

Wood J et. al. Pulmonary Disease in Patients with Marfan Syndrome. *Thorax* (British Medical Journal). 1984 39:780-784.

Berkow R., ed. The Merck Manual-Home Edition.2nd ed. Whitehouse Station, NJ: Merck Research Laboratories; 2003:1608-9.

Channell K. Marfan syndrome. Emedicine Journal http://www.emedicine.com/orthoped/topic414.htm. Updated April 9, 2010. Accessed June 8, 2011.

Chen H. Genetics of Marfan Syndrome. Medscape. http://emedicine.medscape.com/article/946315-overview

Chen H. Marfan syndrome. Emedicine Journal. http://www.emedicine.com/ped/topic1372.htm. Updated March 10, 2010. Accessed June 8, 2011.

Chubb, H & Simpson, J. The use of z-scores in pediatric cardiology. Ann Pediatr Cardiol. 2012 Jul-Dec; 5(2): 179–184.

Cleveland Clinic. Heart Surgery for Marfan Syndrome. http://my.clevelandclinic.org/heart/disorders/aorta_marfan/marfansurgery.aspx

Collod G, Babron M-C, Jondeau G, et al. A second locus for Marfan syndrome maps to chromosome 3p24.2-p25. Nat Genet. 1994;8:264-8.

Conway JE et. al. Marfan syndrome is not associated with intracranial aneurysms. Stroke. 1999 Aug;30(8):1632-6.

Dean JC. Marfan syndrome: clinical diagnosis and management. Eur J Hum Genet. 2007;15:274-33.

Dietz H. Marfan Syndrome. NORD Guide to Rare Disorders. Lippincott Williams & Wilkins. Philadelphia, PA. 2003:218-9.

Dietz HC, Pyeritz RE, Hall BD, et al. The Marfan syndrome caused by a recurrent de novo missense mutation in the fibrillin gene. Nature. 1991;352:337-9.

Dietz HC. Updated 6/30/2009. Marfan Syndrome. In: GeneReviews at GeneTests: Medical Genetics Information Resource (database online). Copyright, University of Washington, Seattle. 1997-2003. Available at http://www.genetests.org. Accessed 6/8/2011.

Disabella E, Grasso M, Marziliano N, Ansaldi S, Lucchelli C, Porcu E, Tagliani M, Pilotto A, Diegoli M, Lanzarini L, Malattia C, Pelliccia A, Ficcadenti A, Gabrielli O, Arbustini E. (2006) Two novel and one known mutation of the TGFβR2 gene in Marfan syndrome not associated with FBN1 gene defects. European Journal of Human Genetics Jan;14(1):34-8.

Forteza A, Cortina JM, Sanchez V, et al. Aortic valve preservation in Marfan syndrome. Initial experience. Rev Esp Cardiol. 2007;60:471-5.

GeneTests Website: www.genetests.org

Jones KL. Ed. Smith's Recognizable Patterns of Human Malformation. 5th ed. W. B. Saunders Co., Philadelphia, PA; 1997:546.

Judge DP, Deitz HC. Marfan's syndrome. Lancet. 2005;366:1965-76.

Gott VL, Cameron DE, Alejo DE, et al. Aortic root replacement in 271 Marfan patients: a 24-year experience. Ann Thorac Surg. 2002;73:438-43.

Le Parc JM, Molcard S Tubach F, et al. Marfan syndrome and fibrillin disorders. Joint Bone Surg. 2000;67:401-7.

Le Parc J-M. Marfan syndrome. Orphanet encyclopedia, February 2005. Available at: http://www.orpha.net/data/patho/GB/Marfan-interm.htm. Accessed June 8, 2011.

Loeys B, De Backer J, Van Acker P, Wettinck K, Pals G, Nuytinck L, Coucke P, De Paepe A (2004) Comprehensive molecular screening of the FBN1 gene favors locus homogeneity of classical Marfan syndrome. Hum Mutat 24:140-6

Loeys BL, Chen J, Neptune ER, Judge DP, Podowski M, Holm T, Meyers J, Leitch CC, Katsanis N, Sharifi N, Xu FL, Myers LA, Spevak PJ, Cameron DE, De Backer J, Hellemans J, Chen Y, Davis EC, Webb CL, Kress W, Coucke P, Rifkin DB, De Paepe AM, Dietz HC (2005) A syndrome of altered cardiovascular, craniofacial, neurocognitive and skeletal development caused by mutations in TGFβR1 or TGFβR2. Nat Genet 37:275-81.

Loeys BL, Dietz HC, Braverman AC, et al. The revised Ghent nosology for the Marfan syndrome. J Med Genet. 2010;47:476-485.

Marfan, Antoine (1896). "Un cas de déformation congénitale des quartre membres, plus prononcée aux extrémitiés, caractérisée par l'allongement des os avec un certain degré d'amincissement" [A case of congenital deformation of the four limbs, more pronounced at the extremities, characterized by elongation of the bones with some degree of thinning].*Bulletins et memoires de la Société medicale des hôspitaux de Paris* **13** (3rd series): 220–226.

Mizuguchi T, Collod-Beroud G, Akiyama T, Abifadel M, Harada N, Morisaki T, Allard D, Varret M, Claustres M, Morisaki H, Ihara M, Kinoshita A, Yoshiura K, Junien C, Kajii T, Jondeau G, Ohta T, Kishino T, Furukawa Y, Nakamura Y, Niikawa N, Boileau C, Matsumoto N. (2004) Heterozygous TGFβR2 mutations in Marfan syndrome. Nature Genetics Aug;36(8):855-60.

Morse et. al. Diagnosis and managemen; -t of infantile marfan syndrome. Pediatrics. 1990. Dec; 86(6):888-95

National Institutes of Health. What is Mitral Valve Prolapse? www.nhlbi.nih.gov/health/health-topics/topics/mvp/

National Institutes of Health: Aneurysm http://www.nhlbi.nih.gov/health/health-topics/topics/arm/livingwith.html. Accessed January 9, 2012.

Neptune, E. What is the appropriate treatment for restrictive lung disease? The Marfan Foundation. https://www.youtube.com/watch?v=0Llw7hfvltM

Online Mendelian Inheritance in Man (OMIM). The Johns Hopkins University. Loeys-Dietz Syndrome, Type 2B; LDS2B (Marfan Syndrome, Type II, Formerly). Entry No: 610380. Last Updated July 6, 2010. Available at: http://www.ncbi.nlm.nih.gov/omim/. Accessed June 8, 2011.

Ramirez F, Dietz HC. Marfan syndrome: from molecular pathogenesis to clinical treatment. Curr Opin Genet Dev. 2007;17:252-8.

Sakai H, Visser R, Ikegawa S, Ito E, Numabe H, Watanabe Y, Mikami H, Kondoh T, Kitoh H, Sugiyama R, Okamoto N, Ogata T, Fodde R, Mizuno S, Takamura K, Egashira M, Sasaki N, Watanabe S, Nishimaki S, Takada F, Nagai T, Okada Y, Aoka Y, Yasuda K, Iwasa M, Kogaki S, Harada N, Mizuguchi T, Matsumoto N. (2006) Comprehensive genetic analysis of relevant four genes in 49 patients with Marfan syndrome or Marfan-related phenotypes. Am J Med Genet A. Aug 15;140(16):1719-25

Sakai LY, Keene DR, Engvall E. Fibrillin, a new 350-kD glycoprotein, is a component of extracellular microfibrils. J Cell Biol. 1986;103:2499-509.

Schievink WI, Parisi JE, Piepgras DG, Michels VV. Intracranial aneurysms in Marfan's syndrome: an autopsy study. *Neurosurgery.*. 1997;41:866–871.

Shores J, Berger KR, Murphy EA and Pyeritz RE. Progression of aortic dilation and the benefit

Singh KK, Rommel K, Mishra A, Karck M, Haverich A, Schmidtke J, Arslan-Kirchner M. (2006) TGFβR1 and TGFβR2 mutations in patients with features of Marfan syndrome and Loeys-Dietz syndrome. Human Mutation Jun 23

Sports Illustrated. Larger than real life. July 04, 2011. http://sportsillustrated.cnn.com/vault/article/magazine/MAG1187806/3/index.htm

Sreeram et. al. Cardiac Abnormalities in the fragile X Syndrome. Br Heart J 1989; 61-289-91.

Weyman, A & Scherrer-Crosbie, M. Marfan syndrome and mitral valve prolapse. *J Clin Invest.* 2004;114(11):1543–1546.

Images
Pectus excavatum: Ahellwig|Wikimedia commons
Aorta: Edorado|Wikimedia Commons
Aortic valve micrograph: Nephron|Wikimedia Commons
FBN1: EMW|Wikimedia Commons
Bunion: Igno2|Wikimedia Commons
Slit Lamp: SchuminWeb| Wikimedia Commons
MVP: Patrick J. Lynch|Wikimedia Commons
Cataract: EyeMD|Wikimedia Commons

Index

abdominal aortic aneurysms, 45
Acromegaly, 97
Acromicric dysplasia, 53
Acute aortic valvular insufficiency, 39
adventitia, 38
amblyopia, 32
amino acid, 17, 20
aneurysm, 10, 22, 23, 41, 42, 43, 44, 45, 46, 47, 54, 91
Angiotensin receptor blockers (ARBs), 73
Anticoagulant medications, 72
aorta, 8, 11, 12, 37, 38, 39, 41, 42, 43, 45, 53, 54, 55, 58, 63, 64, 68, 70, 71, 73
Aortic dilation, 41
aortic dissection, 12, 38, 39, 44, 63, 70, 71, 73, 91, 96
aortic regurgitation, 71
aortic root, 37, 46, 54, 70, 71, 81, 96, 99
aortic root replacement, 37, 81
aortic valve, 37, 39, 46, 70, 98
Aortography, 63
Arachnodactyly, 6, 59

Arteries, 42, 91
astigmatism, 32
Bacterial endocarditis, 40
Beals Syndrome, 22, 95
Bentall procedure, 46
beta-blockers, 12, 83
Bicuspid Aortic Valve, 98
bleb resection, 78
brain aneurysms, 46, 96
Bunions, 31
Calluses, 31
cardiologist, 54, 63
cataract, 36
claw toes, 31
Clinical Trials, 83
composite graft replacement, 46
congestive heart failure, 40
Connective tissue, 7
David Valve-Sparing procedure, 70
de novo, 14, 118
Delayed developmental milestones, 58
Detached retina. *See* retinal detachment
dislocated lens, 33, 34, 58, 74
dissections, 39, 44, 91
Dracon Graft, 72
Dural Ecstasia, 36

dural ectasia, 58, 60
echocardiogram, 60, 70
Ectopia Lentis Syndrome, 23, 95
Ehlers-Danlos Syndrome, 53, 94
Emphysema, 50
Endocarditis prophylaxis, 69
endoscope, 78
endothelial cells, 38
enlarged cornea, 32
enophthalmos, 33
Familial Thoracic Aortic Aneurysm and Dissection, 22, 96
FBN1, 9, 10, 17, 19, 20, 21, 22, 23, 52, 57, 79, 119, 120, 125
fibrillin-1, 9, 19, 20
Fibrillin-1, 9, 19
Flat feet, 31, 75
Flo Hyman, 11
Fragile X Syndrome, 96
genetic mutation, 9
Genetic testing, 21, 24, 57
Genetic Testing, 21
germline mutations, 14
Ghent criteria, 54
Gigantism, 97
glaucoma, 33, 59
hemorrhage, 39, 82
highly arched palate, 27, 95
Homocystinuria, 22
Homograft technique, 71
Hunched back. See Kyphosis
Hyperpituitarism, 97

Hyperthyroidism, 97
intima, 38
Klinefelter Syndrome, 98
Kyphosis, 30
ligaments, 19, 27, 29, 31, 58
Loeys-Dietz Syndrome, 23, 91, 92, 93, 119
losartan, 73
MASS Phenotype, 23, 98
MASS syndrome, 53, 99
media, 38
medical geneticist, 54
microfibrils, 19, 118
Missense mutations, 17
Mitral insufficiency, 40
mitral regurgitation, 71
Mitral valve prolapse, 22, 23, 48
MRI, 60, 62, 63
myopia, 23, 32, 55, 95
Myopia, 74
nearsightedness. *See* myopia
ocular, 7
pectus excavatum, 41, 58, 99
Pectus excavatum, 28, 76, 92, 125
Pericardial tamponade, 40
physical activity, 68, 69
pleurodesis, 78
Pneumothorax, 78
Pregnancy, 79
Protrusio acetabuli, 73
Restrictive Lung Disease, 48

retinal detachment, 33, 34, 75, 100
Schprintzen-Goldberg Syndrome, 99
scoliosis, 30, 55, 60, 75, 76, 89, 96, 99, 100
Scoliosis, 29, 59, 75, 76, 89
Shprintzen-Goldberg syndrome, 53
Shprintzen-Goldberg Syndrome, 23
Sleep apnea, 51
slit-lamp eye examination, 34
Small in-frame deletions, 17
somatic mutation, 15
Spontaneous Pneumothorax, 49
Stickler Syndrome, 24, 100
Stiff skin syndrome, 53
stretch marks, 55, 99

TGF-β, 9
TGFβR2, 10, 21, 119, 120, 121, 122, 123, 124, 125
thoracic aortic aneurysm, 8, 43, 44
thoracoscopy, 78
Thumb sign, 56
transesophageal echocardiography, 60
transforming growth factor beta, 9, 19
Transforming Growth Factor-Beta Receptor, 10
Turned ankles, 31
Vascular Ehlers-Danlos Syndrome, 22
Warfarin, 72, 82
Weill-Marchesani syndrome, 52
Yacoub remodeling, 71
Z-scores, 41

Printed in Great Britain
by Amazon